The Itch

The Itch

Scabies

ERROL CRAIG, MD, PhD

Clinical Dermatologist, The Permanente Medical Group, Inc.
Walnut Creek, California, USA

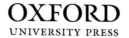

OXFORD
UNIVERSITY PRESS

OXFORD
UNIVERSITY PRESS

Great Clarendon Street, Oxford, OX2 6DP,
United Kingdom

Oxford University Press is a department of the University of Oxford.
It furthers the University's objective of excellence in research, scholarship,
and education by publishing worldwide. Oxford is a registered trade mark of
Oxford University Press in the UK and in certain other countries

© Oxford University Press 2022

The moral rights of the author have been asserted

First Edition published in 2022

Published in the United States of America by Oxford University Press
198 Madison Avenue, New York, NY 10016, United States of America

British Library Cataloguing in Publication Data

Data available

Library of Congress Control Number: 2021950475

ISBN 978–0–19–284840–6

DOI: 10.1093/med/9780192848406.001.0001

Printed and bound by
CPI Group (UK) Ltd, Croydon, CR0 4YY

To Nahide and George

The author would like to thank the following individuals for their encouragement, comments, and critical review of the manuscript: Aileen Chang, Margaret DeLacy, Ken Katz, Lisa Rasmussen, Ross Jackson, Kati Clyman, Yasmin Vitalius, Nahide Craig, George Craig, and Erica Pacheco. Nicole Bonino and Daniele Carsano provided assistance with Italian translation. The author expresses gratitude to the librarians at Kaiser Permanente for their assistance in my relentless requests to obtain documents. Additional thanks: Kevin Carney (Friedman bookplate), Simon Heilesen and Alex Mellanby (historical photos), Angelica Wouters (mite identification), and the team at Oxford University Press.

Names of patients have been changed and clinical details may have been modified to protect patient privacy.

All attempts have been made to ensure accuracy of information, and any errors that may exist are solely my own.

Contents

1. Introduction   1

2. Transmissibility   5

3. The Rash   23

4. The Mite   55

5. Epidemiology   73

6. History   93

7. Early Pioneers   121

8. Therapy   135

9. Conclusion   161

References   163
Index   173

It may be objected that considerable ink has been wasted in retelling such an oft old tale as scabies. But while trite and commonplace, dull and sordid, it nevertheless assumes commanding importance, when unidentified and uncontrolled.

—William Cunningham MD, 1915. (105)

1

Introduction

As a newly minted doctor at the ripe age of 35, I found myself sitting in a nook of the dermatology clinic with my white coat on, feeling vaguely puzzled. I was in the midst of my dermatology residency training, and had arrived at clinic a few minutes prior, having spent the morning in lectures elsewhere. To my left and right were patient exam rooms. Around me were chairs for dermatology residents, medical students, and the more senior doctors to sit and discuss cases. At our disposal were several computers, as well as a wall full of serious dermatological tomes, some running more than a thousand pages in length. While waiting for my first patient to be roomed, I noticed something unusual about the nearest exam room. The door was not only shut, but additionally blocked off by a flimsy criss-cross of blue masking tape running from corner to corner of the door frame. Where the strands crossed each other in the middle was affixed a small yellow sticky note with the words 'HOUSEKEEPING' scribbled on it, all in capitals. What could possibly be going on?

It appears that while I had been out for the morning, a case of scabies had befallen the clinic, with repercussions now lasting into the afternoon. And just what exactly had taken an exam room out of commission? Scabies is an itchy contagious skin disease caused by the scabies mite, which resides in the skin and can only just barely be detected by the naked eye, provided one has exceptional eyesight (7). The intensely itchy rash that it causes, can be at times tricky to diagnose, but with a little bit of luck, and patience, it is actually possible with a fine blade to extract the mite out of the skin and examine it under the microscope. Here one can see the human itch mite *Sarcoptes scabiei* in its full glory— fat and pudgy, with weird spikes and long running spines. It has been likened to a tortoise, but to my eye, it looks more like a comically obese blob.

To those who have never been afflicted or perhaps have never even heard of scabies, it might seem but a medical curiosity. Who would believe that a tiny male mite would exist that seeks out and impregnates a similarly tiny female mite that then proceeds to lay eggs which hatch and form baby mites, all in your skin? And that this could lead to a skin disease and an intense itch? At first, it may be perceived only subtly, or in fact not at all.[1] With time it leads to fits of scratching, where its symptoms can be disturbingly out of proportion to any physical findings. Patients can feel like they are losing their mind. The Itch can distract from work and study, and severely disrupt sleep. Often patients will scratch their skin so heavily that they develop skin infections on top of their already miserable rash.

Having sensed that I missed all the action, I sought out the medical assistant from the morning. 'You can't use that room, you know that right?' she blurted at me before I could get a word in edgewise. When I expressed regret that I wasn't around for the excitement, she replied, 'Ha! Are you joking? It's so creepy', adding, 'I'm itchy and I washed my hands five times already.' And off she went. Here was a dermatological disease which elicited a strong sentiment, and it prompted me to ask myself: What do we really know about this disease? How contagious is it really? A curious look at a few of the reference textbooks provided lots of details, but didn't really address my questions. This one chance event in clinic prompted me into digging a little bit deeper into the topic of scabies.

And what I found is that the story of scabies is a fascinating one, which has preoccupied patients and physicians alike for millennia. Colloquially known as simply 'The Itch', scabies is a disease rich in history. The presence of a mite associated with The Itch has been known for hundreds, perhaps even thousands of years. Yet ironically, the dogma of medical antiquity prevented this knowledge from being properly digested. Only slowly and begrudgingly as medieval concepts have been shed and rational scientific thought adopted, has our modern concept of scabies emerged. This book details the long and meandering path taken by scabies, no pun intended, from insufferable itch to readily treatable medical ectoparasite.

Along the way physicians are exposed as being hopelessly backward. Poisons and other ineffectual remedies are enthusiastically dispensed, resulting in much misery. Lay healers and those with no formal medical education, relying strictly on the power of observation, ironically provide the most help treating the sick. Early pioneers are ridiculed, and authorities—academic, medical, and even the Church—take a stand when ideas become too modern and progressive. Finally, amid much academic controversy, the evidence becomes overwhelming. And in the end, we have the first convincing scientific description of an infectious disease. Not bad—hey you've come a long way scaby!

In spite of the fact that we now know the cause of scabies and have the tools to treat and cure, the modern experience of The Itch can still be miserable. It is difficult to diagnose and not uncommon for patients to be mistakenly given a variety of ineffectual salves and balms. To those who are familiar with or have had scabies, even the thought of it can cause hair on the back of the neck to stand up. I suspect for you this book will represent a spooky and somewhat obsessive read.

In these pages, I shall strive to assimilate the historical writings and more modern investigations on scabies while weaving in anecdotes from my own clinical career. My goal is to demystify scabies and explore what we do and do not know about this arthropod, parasite, and general pest. My experiences have taught me to respect scabies as a disease and not to underestimate it, but also not to fear it. And if nothing else, I hope to reassure that it is far less contagious than, at least, was conveyed to me when I was starting my training. And this I have learned through my readings but also confirmed from personal experience.

Note

1. James (VI) King of Scotland, and later England, was reported to have said that 'None but kings and princes should have The Itch for the sensation of scratching was so delightful' (127). In my experience, few sufferers of scabies would agree with this description.

2

Transmissibility

Gertrude

Fast forward many years to my clinical practice. I would be seeing Gertrude today, whom I had seen once previously, when I removed a few cancerous growths from her arms that had seen the better of 90 years of sun. I remember her mainly by the intense pain I appeared to cause in the process of anaesthetising her lesions. Patients have varying levels of pain tolerance ranging from those who never even flinch, to those for whom the lightest touch can elicit shrieks and howls. Gertrude was firmly in the latter camp. When I heard that she'd be coming back to see me I suspected it would be another most unpleasant experience for her.

And it was, poor Gertrude. She arrived from her assisted-living facility in a taxi with her caregiver Jan. The first inkling of a problem was when I heard from the clinic staff that she would be late. Why? Because she was in the parking lot unable get out of the taxi. Physically she was stuck. 'Hmmm, let me see what's going on', I muttered as I headed outside to check on the situation. I spotted Jan in the lobby and followed her back to the car, thinking I might even be able to assess and treat Gertrude then and there. Sure enough, there she was sitting in the back seat of the cab, whimpering and frazzled. Her back hurt, and her legs were too weak to swing out of the car. She weighed too much to be lifted out easily. 'How did she even get in the taxi in the first place?' I wondered to myself. Jan and I spent a few minutes conferring with her and trying to figure out what to do; meanwhile the cab driver looked most annoyed, the time-is-money society that we live in seemingly robbing him of any compassion.

We decided that we would physically assist her out of the cab. A wheelchair was positioned adjacent to the car. I entered the back seat and scooted up close to her. 'Gertrude, I will hold you and prop up your back while your caregiver grabs your hips, and we'll glide you into the wheelchair.' 'Ok', she feebly mumbled. I reached under her arms, giving her a bear hug, embracing her upper torso, while Jan tried to nudge her out of the car. 'My legs, my legs', she cried, 'they won't hold me.' 'Ok, grab my hands', I suggested, 'and Jan will support your waist while we gently slide you to the wheelchair.' She grasped my hands but quickly balked. 'No I can't, please help me.' Gertrude was in full-out panic mode, weak and seemingly stuck in a taxi, while Jan and I went through various possibilities on how to extract her safely.

After several minutes of this and an even further exasperated taxi driver hovering in the background, our clinic manager showed up with a piece of professional transport equipment resembling a toddler chair swing with multiple straps attached to a winch-like apparatus. Within a few minutes we had Gertrude strapped in and hoisted out of the cab, transferred to the wheelchair, and whisked into the clinic.

Once in the exam room, she calmed down a little and apologized for the trouble she had caused. By all means it was the start of an unusual clinic visit. 'No problem, Gertrude. I'm sorry you had to go through all that. So let's see what brings you in....' She related that she was extremely itchy. She extended her arms out and showed me her hands, which revealed dozens of small zig-zag white and flaky patterned lines most prominently where the base of her thumb and index finger met the skin of her palm. In a way it looked like a bizarre pattern of peeling, or perhaps even air blisters. Yet I knew immediately here were burrows, the cavernous tracks of scabies and its tell-tale sign. At times one of the most difficult diagnoses to make, and at times one of the easiest, this was a slam dunk case of scabies, straight out of the textbook. I told her she had scabies, and could not help but catching site of her caregiver Jan glaring at me with mouth open. My medical assistant also peered at me, though a bit less conspicuously. The contagious nature of the disease had them worried, and the tension in the air was palpable. 'Well let me take a scraping to look at under the microscope', I added almost out of routine. Seeing is believing, and is of great utility in less straightforward cases; here I had no doubt. Yet I faithfully donned my purple nitrile gloves and took her hand. In my other hand was my dermatoscope, a small magnifying optical apparatus with a powerful polarized light source, and a filter to subtract out scattered or incident light. I localized the end of a burrow and peering through the dermatoscope saw a minute triangular structure corresponding to the pigmented mouth parts and front legs of the scabies mite. With a very sharp blade, I surgically plucked an ever so small piece of skin including this fragment, transferred it to a glass slide, and headed over to the microscope. There as expected, I saw the pudgy oval body of the scabies mite with its stubby legs terminating in long spines.

When I came back to inform Gertrude, it dawned on me that but 20 minutes earlier I had my arms fully around her, holding her at first by her arms and then by her hands, trying to assist her out of the taxi. Would this be the beginning of my contracting scabies? For her caregiver and other nursing home residents, this was in fact a very legitimate question, as scabies is contagious and can spread to close contacts. But having been a student of scabies for some while, I was not worried for myself; limited contact is not typically how scabies spreads. And I felt quite confident in this knowledge, being familiar with a very unique set of human experiments that were performed in World War II England by an entomologist named Kenneth Mellanby (1908–1993) (Figure 2.1).

Mellanby

Scabies has a long and intriguing history, dating back to antiquity. At the risk of presenting a jumbled chronology, however, let us first jump to the middle of the twentieth century to discuss the life and work of Mellanby. Mellanby

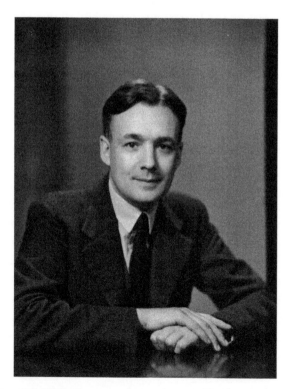

Figure 2.1 Kenneth Mellanby, exact date unknown, likely just prior to or at the very beginning years of his pioneering scabies investigations.
Courtesy of Alex Mellanby.

undertook a most remarkable series of human experiments that forever changed our understanding of scabies, in particular, how it is spread or transmitted. Where Mellanby enters the story, the scabies mite had already been long discovered and was known to be the causative agent of scabies. Moreover effective treatment existed. Yet scabies as a disease was imperfectly understood. The lifecycle of the mite had been studied, but much misinformation was still present. Scabies, moreover, was not regarded as a problem of medical importance. The medical community mainly viewed it as a nuisance, not meriting in-depth study. In fact, Mellanby did even not set out to work on scabies initially. As often happens in history, a unique set of circumstances led him to stumble onto the subject. The storm clouds of World War II sucked him in.

Mellanby trained at King's College, Cambridge, studying bugs, or more formally the branch of science called entomology. In 1929 he worked as a researcher at the London School of Hygiene and Tropical Medicine (Figure 2.2). At the outbreak of the second World War, Mellanby held the Sorby Research Fellowship of the Royal Society, working at the University of Sheffield. When it became clear that war in Europe was inevitable, a wave of patriotic spirit engulfed the United Kingdom. Mellanby decided he wanted to utilize his scientific knowledge to contribute to his country's war effort. He petitioned the health and military authorities for suggestions of pressing medical problems to study, but was given little encouragement or guidance.[1] Mellanby thus decided to set aside his prior work on insect physiology and devote himself to the study of human lice.

As had been clearly demonstrated in the first World War, human lice constituted a major medical problem in the military theatre. Aside from incapacitating soldiers, lice were known disease carriers of typhus and trench fever. These diseases alone were responsible for millions of deaths in the grimy, unhygienic, and cramped conditions that characterized the trench warfare of World War I, a time when antibiotics had yet to be discovered. Mellanby chose to investigate head lice, which had been noted in high numbers amongst children transferred to the English countryside with the expectation of upcoming urban air raids. In his discussion with medical officers and physicians, however, he quickly realized that scabies was perhaps an even bigger problem. In particular there was concern that with upcoming air raids, scabies might spread like wildfire in crowded underground air shelters.

Intrigued, Mellanby immersed himself in reviewing all that was known about scabies. Certainly there was no shortage of information. The trick, however, was to separate out fact from fiction. To gain a solid basis for his knowledge, Mellanby was directed by colleague A. M. H. Gray to study the

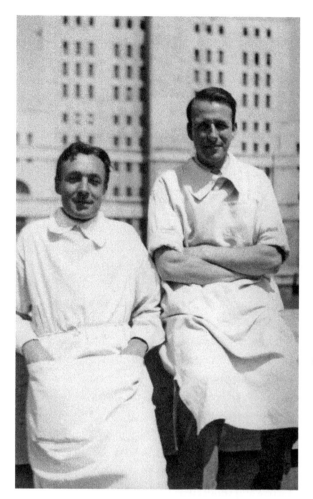

Figure 2.2 Kenneth Mellanby (1908–1993) (L) standing next to Bjørn Heilesen (1913–2000) (R) on the roof of London School of Hygiene and Tropical Medicine, 1947. This photo was taken several years after Mellanby's ground-breaking studies of scabies.
Courtesy of Simon Heilesen.

classic works of Ferdinand Ritter von Hebra, the famous nineteenth-century Viennese dermatologist and authority on scabies.[2] Mellanby immediately recognized that important voids existed in the knowledge of the scabies lifecycle, particularly in how it was transmitted from one individual to another. At the time, there were many different theories; scabies was variably considered to be a disorder of uncleanliness, a venereal disease, a disease of the military, or a disorder of crowding and close contact.

The prevalence of scabies dramatically shot up during the course of the second World War, much as it had done during the first World War. It is estimated that between 1 and 2 million individuals in the British Isles alone were infested with scabies by the early 1940s (19). Depending on wartime circumstances, the civilian population might regard scabies as but an itchy nuisance, and perhaps the least of their problems. For the military however, it was an entirely different matter. As was clearly seen during the first World War, The Itch could relegate men to the sick barracks and render units incapable of being effective fighting forces. The military mentality was 'every man incapacitated from duty—it matters not by what means—is a gain to the enemy' (23).[3] Thus Mellanby recognized that understanding the details of how scabies was transmitted, in addition to having medical importance, could also have military implications. He approached the problem of scabies by assuming blankets and garments were mainly at fault for spreading the disease:

> I must make it clear that at the outset the problem which appeared to me of paramount importance was that of transmission, that is to say, just how and where did the uninfected person pick up the scabies mite and so 'catch' the disease. I believed, with most others, that infection usually took place through the medium of inanimate objects, i.e. mites that were to be found lurking in dirty blankets waiting to infect the unfortunate individual who used them next. I was even prepared to believe that the scabies epidemic which was apparent in these early days of the war was mainly due to the military, for soldiers were, I thought, being infected by the bedding which was not being frequently enough disinfested, and so they were then taking home the disease to infect their wives and children when on leave. (19)

Studying how scabies is transmitted had been, and still is, fraught with logistical and ethical difficulties. Mellanby fortuitously benefitted from wartime circumstances. He found himself in a climate where there existed a willing and eager group of experimental subjects amongst conscientious objectors to the war. In 1939, the British Parliament had passed the National Service (Armed Forces) Act, which mandated widespread military conscription, but made provisions for conscientious objectors. Such objectors could avoid conscription, in return for performing noncombatant jobs. Yet the truly principled objector did not want to engage in noncombatant military projects. However, they might be willing to make a contribution, even at some discomfort to themselves, should their participation provide broader benefits for humanity, including allowing themselves to be subject to medical experimentation. Mellanby wrote:

The idea of using conscientious objectors had been growing in my mind for some time, and I knew that at this time there were many individuals who felt they could not take part in the war as combatants and who at the same time wished to serve humanity. In the summer of 1940, the number of outlets for such service was small, and many pacifists appeared to think that the duties which they were performing, or to which they had been directed, were very unimportant. (19)

With the encouragement of colleagues, Mellanby wrote a proposal to the Ministry of Health for the study of scabies using human volunteers, specifically conscientious objectors, in coordination with the army medical staff. To his surprise, his proposal was quickly approved.[4]

As the German air force, the Luftwaffe, stepped up its bombing campaign of the English heartland, Mellanby set about establishing his scabies research institute. He procured a Victorian villa at 18 Oakholme Road, which became known as 'Fairholmes', in the Broomhill suburb of Sheffield, an industrial town in central England (Figure 2.3).

He set about furnishing it with towels, bedding, and, to keep costs low, used furniture. In December, Sheffield itself was subject to a German blitz, though his budding institute came out rather unscathed with damage being mostly in the form of broken windows. Under the menacing conditions of war, Mellanby gathered up, with the help of local pacifist organizations, a dozen conscientious objectors. Included in this group were individuals from different walks of life, including an electrician, a milkman, a shop assistant, a ladies hairdresser, a clerk, and a baker. The goal was to use these human volunteers to better understand the natural history of scabies.

Initial experiments were set up to demonstrate the conditions under which scabies could be transmitted from soiled blankets and clothing. Accepting the dogma that blankets and other items would have to be disinfected to prevent transmission, sterilization equipment in the form of a large, heated cupboard was constructed. Volunteers were asked to sleep naked amongst 'infected blankets' of scabietic soldiers, and were also made to wear the clothing of scabies-infested soldiers—vests, pants, shirts, and trousers, day and night, for at least a week. An amused Mellanby described the scene: 'Not infrequently one saw a pacifist volunteer, who had refused to wear uniform or join the army, clad almost entirely in khaki garments and wearing them with good grace.' On a routine basis subjects would then strip naked and submit themselves to scrutiny from head to toe, whereby Mellanby and colleagues would examine 'every square inch of their skin' with a hand lens or binocular microscope. To

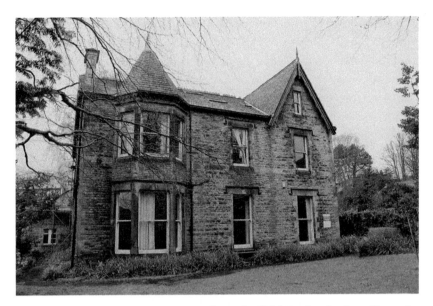

Figure 2.3 Fairholmes, the Victorian villa in Sheffield, England, where Kenneth Mellanby conducted his studies on scabies during World War II.
Courtesy of John Broom.

everyone's surprise, as Mellanby wrote, scabies did not seem to be as highly contagious as anticipated:

> I had assumed that as a result of the type of exposure ... within a few days of using the bedding or clothing normal clinical scabies would be apparent in the majority of the volunteers. Therefore no one was more surprised than I when weeks and months, covered by a very large number of different experiments of this kind, went by, and not one of my volunteers had developed scabies. It seemed obvious that the current views on transmission were somehow at fault, and it was necessary entirely to change the whole plan of the experiments. The reactions of the volunteers at this time were interesting. At the outset they were all naturally a bit nervous about what was going to happen to them. They had volunteered to have scabies, and were all perfectly willing to go through with it but it was going to be an unpleasant experience. But now that they had been doing the work of volunteers for what seemed a very long period, and no one had developed the disease or had anything unpleasant to report—they began to feel a bit fraudulent and all became exceedingly keen to develop and suffer from the disease.

We seemed unable to infect any of our volunteers, which made it difficult to test out other types of transmission. I considered all manner of desperate possibilities. Would it be practicable to ask a pacific volunteer and an infected soldier to share a bed, to see if transmission took place? And would it be possible to test out the venereal hypothesis? We discussed whether we should try to find some accommodating young woman with scabies to use as a source of infection. My volunteers became, I gather, a bit worried that they would be asked to commit adultery in the interests of science, and I was worried that if such an experiment were to take place the police might raid the Institute and I would be arrested for keeping a 'disorderly house'. (19)

Mellanby did not have to resort to such measures, and eventually was able to demonstrate the transmission of scabies from one individual to another. However it wound up being much more difficult than he had originally thought. Simply sleeping in a bed previously used by a known scabies sufferer was not sufficient to spread the disease—of 19 volunteers who did so, none contracted scabies. The first cases of transmission were only detected when volunteers donned the well-worn underwear of scabies sufferers while still warm—and of the 32 volunteers who obliged, only 2 contracted scabies. Moreover, it took a long time for scabies to develop in his volunteer subjects. Instead of manifesting in hours or days, as he had assumed, Mellanby found that that it took roughly 6 weeks for volunteers to develop The Itch. Mellanby described similar results based on experiments he performed on himself:

My own experience was typical. I allowed a mite to burrow into my own wrist, and observed it—almost like a pet—for two months. Each day the tunnel was enlarged, eggs were located in the burrow, but I have no skin reaction. It was only in the fifth week that a redness was observed around the mite, and that skin irritation became obvious. (2)

Once Mellanby had achieved success in spreading scabies, he set about to systematically study it. Infested individuals were left untreated for up to 9 months, and carefully observed. Mellanby found that the tell-tale lesion of scabies, the meandering burrow, was actually present in an uninflamed state well before the 6-week mark when his subjects would begin to experience itching or discomfort. Slowly with time, newly infested volunteers with burrows started to develop symptoms, an immunological process known as sensitization. Approximately 6 weeks after infestation, most subjects experienced severe itch, often significant enough to cause sleep disruption. Mellanby wrote about his subject's experiences:

> The experiment was very unpleasant for the participants. They had, many of them, in the first experiments been infected for a few weeks only and they felt rather that the symptoms of 'intolerable irritation' and other unpleasant experiences attributed in the literature to clinical scabies tended to be exaggerated. They soon changed their minds. After being infected for about a hundred days they mostly agreed that what they had previously experienced was negligible. Some kept rough brushes to rub over the skin to relieve irritation. On cold nights some would rise from a sleepless bed and walk naked through the house, as when the skin was chilled the itching temporarily subsided and sometimes, if sufficiently tired, it was possible to fall asleep before the skin got warm and the irritation returned. Certain volunteers were reduced to sleeping naked as they scratched so vigorously in their sleep that their pyjamas were torn to shreds. (19)[5]

Interestingly, Mellanby found that the time to contract scabies differed depending on whether it was an initial or repeat exposure. He showed that subjects who were previously infected, treated, and cured of their scabies developed itch and discomfort within 24 hours after reinfestation, rather than slowly over 6 weeks. The reason for this, he proposed, was that previously infected patients were already sensitized and did not require weeks to develop an immunological reaction to the mite. He experimentally demonstrated the phenomenon of sensitization by injecting crushed mite extracts into the skin of volunteers.[6] In healthy controls and those who had scabies less than 3 months, injection of mite extracts caused no effect. However in subjects who had been infested with scabies for at least 6 months, injection of mite extracts caused an inflammatory response within 24–36 hours, which Mellanby described as 'a wheal the size of a sixpence' (58).[7]

Mellanby further investigated the mechanism by which scabies spreads from one individual to another. To do so, he performed a series of mite transplantation experiments. He found that he was able to spread scabies by physically plucking out a female mite from an infested individual and implanting her on one of his uninfected volunteers. Scabies could not similarly be spread through the transfer of eggs or immature mites.[8] Mellanby thus concluded that it was the female mite that was responsible for the spread of scabies.

In addition to his studies on experimental subjects, Mellanby launched a 30-bed scabies hospital where he treated soldiers with the standard soak, scrub, and sulphur treatment, as well as an all-female scabies-treatment facility staffed entirely by women. He taught military authorities, including Canadian personnel, how to identify scabies, holding small informal courses for them. Roughly one in four cases sent to him wound up being a skin disorder other than scabies, which he immediately passed on to the Dermatology Department at the Sheffield Royal Infirmary. 'We did not pretend to be able to diagnose or treat other skin diseases than scabies', he wrote. From his experiences he soon became a master scabies diagnostician (190). Mellanby later described his technique, which required magnification, good lighting, and scrupulous examination:

> The procedure is as follows: The patient lies naked on a couch in a good light in a warm room and the surface of the body is inspected, using a watchmaker's eyeglass; the mites are extracted with a mounted needle. With a little experience it is possible to detect the mites in the skin before removal. Each patient is carefully examined at least two, and often more, times, and the accuracy of the results has been ensured by keeping some patients from whom the mites have been removed in this way under observation for periods of weeks, to ensure that none has been missed. (76)

Following this protocol, Mellanby was able to compile a listing of how many female mites could be found on each and every individual examined, which he referred to as the 'parasite rate' (76).[9]

In all, Mellanby removed 9978 female mites from a total of 886 male patients, an average of 11 female mites per patient. Far from teeming with them, the average infested individual harboured less than a dozen scabies mites! This statistic helps one understand how a doctor may easily miss the diagnosis of scabies after only a quick or cursory examination.

Based on his surprising findings of low mite burden and limited transmissibility, Mellanby suggested that the average scabies-infested individual was far less contagious than many had assumed. He indirectly observed this fact by noting that for most of the course of his experiments, no staff or visitors accidentally contracted scabies. Only later, when several of his subjects harboured mites in the hundreds, did accidental infection occur.[10] Mellanby thus proposed that only the small subset of patients with a very high mite burden were likely to be contagious through casual contact. But because the great majority of patients bear very few mites, he concluded that overall scabies is not a highly contagious disease. Thus, with Mellanby's data in the back of my mind, I wasn't particularly worried that I would catch scabies from Gertrude.

Mellanby also performed experiments to dispel the notion of scabies as a disorder of uncleanliness, or 'dirt disease'. He took uninfected volunteers and divided them into two groups—one which bathed daily and other which rarely bathed. While he found the examination of the latter group disagreeable, overall both groups were equal in their ability to transmit scabies to others.[11] Mellanby thus put to rest the theory that catching or passing along scabies had anything to do with cleanliness.

Mellanby immediately recognized there were practical implications to his finding that scabies was difficult to experimentally transmit. It meant that attention and resources need not be wasted on disinfecting or discarding clothing, blankets, and other personal items that a scabies patient had recently used. In fact, von Hebra had come to a similar conclusion nearly a century prior, though firmly ingrained beliefs on this topic meant that his recommendations were largely overlooked. Mellanby showed that all scabies patients who underwent treatment relapsed at the same rate, irrespective of whether their belongings were disinfested or not. We now know the reason why it is not necessary to kill scabies mites on inanimate objects—for the most part they die on their own. The scabies mite is not a hearty creature, and under most conditions, those mites removed from the human skin for longer than 24 hours dry out, shrivel up, and die.

Based on Mellanby's data and observations, the Ministry of Health officially adopted the policy that disinfestation of bedding and belongings was not required to properly treat scabies. Resources would be better spent tracking down and treating family and other close contacts. Re-exposure to rare mites which came from bedding or clothing that happened to retain infectious potential would be of no consequence for, as they put it: 'sufficient medicament persists on the skin for a good many hours to kill any parasites with which it comes in contact and garments which may be infectious are rendered innocuous'. Moreover, in the unlikely circumstance of reinfestation, retreatment would be preferable to expending labour and material on routine disinfestation.

Mellanby thus put the issue of disinfection to rest. As he had originally hoped for, his conclusions proved to have important military implications, freeing up resources on the battlefield. Skipping the arduous disinfection process, termed 'stoving', in 1943 alone was estimated to save the military £500,000. Mellanby's research thus represented a handsome investment on the roughly £5000 that it cost the Ministry of Health. Based on this work, the Ministry of Health made and distributed an informational film on scabies for doctor, nurses, and others involved in the diagnosis or treatment of scabies. From these investigations in Sheffield, Mellanby was able make fundamental insights into the transmission, treatment, and immunology of scabies. His conclusions continue to have practical importance and inform our understanding of scabies to this day.

Encouraged by the fruits of his investigations, Mellanby and his volunteer subjects proceeded to investigate an entirely different subject. With governmental approval, he designed experiments to determine the hydration and energy needs of shipwrecked persons. His volunteers submitted themselves to various lengths of fasting and water restriction, followed by medical examination and laboratory testing. Here, Mellanby was also able to draw important conclusions to aid the war effort. Based on his experiments, Mellanby determined that lifeboat supplies should contain larger quantities of water at the expense of food. He then proceeded to study the role of vitamin deprivation in his volunteers (Figure 2.4).

Of particular interest was the minimum amount of vitamin A that humans could consume and still maintain proper health. These experiments, which

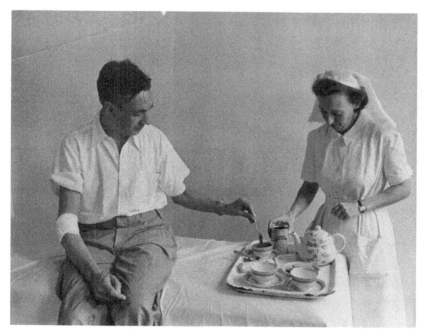

Figure 2.4 Kenneth Mellanby, exact date unknown, being served tea after appearing to have blood drawn. Toward the end of his scabies investigations, Mellanby participated in a series of vitamin-depravation experiments, which would have entailed testing of various body fluids, including blood. Thus this photo likely dates to 1944 or 1945.
Courtesy of Alex Mellanby.

wound up lasting several years, involved the strict measurement and analysis of all dietary intake as well as output including excrement. This work was undertaken with colleagues from Sheffield, including the famous biochemist Sir Hans Krebs.[12] Subsequent experiments on vitamin C deprivation were performed during the late war years at the Sorby Institute, though not under Mellanby's auspices. As the years rolled on, vitamin deprivation experiments came to require all of the institute's resources, and scabies experiments were phased out (41).

Mellanby's research with volunteer subjects was performed during extraordinary times:

> I did not know quite what I was letting my volunteers in for when I originally asked them to submit to infection with scabies. I knew the disease could be very unpleasant and had heard patients saying that the intolerable itching had prevented them from sleeping for weeks, but it seemed unlikely that any permanent harm would be done to any of the volunteers. Nevertheless, at the outset I imagined that it would be a necessary safeguard for each man to sign some sort of detailed contract, setting forth his duties and the risks he was taking.... (19)

Eschewing formality, Mellanby, ultimately decided to forgo any sort of legalistic contract. He took pains to point out that his subjects were true volunteers, who had the right to terminate their participation, an assertion that has been questioned by modern day ethicists.[13] Mellanby specifically wrote that he opposed research being carried out on unwilling subjects such as prisoners, or others in a disadvantaged position who had been bribed. He concluded his thoughts with the ominous observation: 'The way in which things have developed in Germany should serve as a warning'.

Ultimately, the horror of the Nazi experimentation on concentration camp victims, as well as other World War II atrocities, would lead to the development of standards for human experimentation. These were first laid out in the Nuremberg code (1947), and then more broadly detailed as a code of medical ethics in the Declaration of Geneva (1948). Subsequently, the Declaration of Helsinki (1975) has built upon these and has been continuously modified and updated to deal more broadly with the ethics of modern clinical research. By current standards, Mellanby's experiments would in fact be regarded as unethical.[14] And thus, in this day and age, similar calibre human experimentation on scabies or any other disease for that matter is unlikely to be repeated (Figure 2.5).

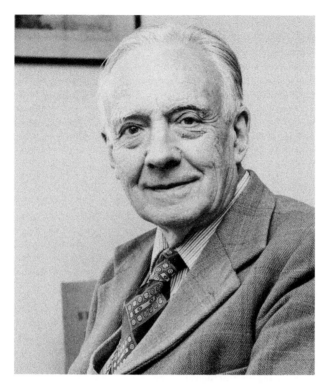

Figure 2.5 Kenneth Mellanby, Officer of the Order of the British Empire, in his more mature years.
Courtesy of the Archives of the University of Sheffield.

Notes

1. As Mellanby would later write, 'It was evident that any initiative would have to come from me' (108).
2. Mellanby wrote:
   > Among the mass of writing about scabies there were to be found lucid accounts of first-class work, but unless one had made a particular study of the subject it was almost impossible to sift these from a mass of indifferent and inaccurate papers. Thus the great Viennese dermatologist Hebra discovered almost all the main facts about scabies a hundred years ago, and if proper reliance had been placed on his results, instead of their being practically forgotten and displaced by inaccurate information based often on the study of unrelated parasites attacking animals and not man, a great deal of human suffering would have been avoided.
3. British soldiers disabled by scabies and its complications were a significant problem in World War I with the average hospital stay due secondary infections being over 1 month.
4. Mellanby wrote that he, 'was not too sanguine that it would appear practicable to the [Health] Ministry or Treasury', yet his proposal was approved with only mild bureaucratic delay. 'I do not think that "red tape" was allowed to cause any real delay', he wrote,

'... as these discussions were being carried out when the Ministry and most people in London were greatly preoccupied by German air raids' (19).

5. Norman Proctor was a baker prior to the war and volunteered for service with Mellanby at the Sorby research institute. He recalled:

> It was extremely itchy. At night the men would get out of bed and walk around naked in the cold to stop the itching. The cure in the early days was awful. Another volunteer held you down in a very hot bath, then they rubbed you with sulphur ointment. It caused impetigo and other skin troubles. Later Dr Mellanby treated us with Benzyl Benzoate. My five mites had multiplied to 59 before they were cleared off. They were all over my body. (41)

6. This process is similar to how today exposure to tuberculosis is tested for in many medical settings. Mycobacterial tuberculosis antigens, in the form of purified protein derivative, are injected into dermis of a patient's forearm, and the injection site is subsequently monitored for the development of a wheal.

7. This process is known as delayed type hypersensitivity, and is one of the mechanisms that our immune system utilizes to defend our bodies from pathogens and external agents.

8. Mellanby wrote:

> On six occasions batches of eggs numbering from three to twenty were removed from the burrows on cases of scabies and placed on the skin of uninfected volunteers. The eggs were kept in position by a small ring of vulcanite and protected by a bandage until they hatched. In none of these cases was an infection produced. Numbers of larvae were also transferred on seven occasions, and in no case was an infection established ... Adult female parasites were removed from patients and placed on the body of the volunteer. In every case where this was done to an individual who had never before been infected with the disease provided that no treatment was given, then typical clinical scabies developed eventually. (58)

9. Mellanby wrote, 'With experience it is possible to discover-and to remove-every burrowing adult female mite on a patient' (2). Of note Mellanby was only detecting mites present in burrows, which are strictly female mites. Male mites tend to localize in or around hair follicles and roam the surface of the skin freely and are thus not readily detected by this technique.

10. Here, Mellanby clearly demonstrated that occasional individuals can be highly contagious.

> For a period of 18 months, when as a rule more than half of a total household of twenty persons was infected, with most individuals showing parasitic infections higher than the average but not higher than 50, no infection of 'controls' or of visitors who mixed freely with the infected volunteers, took place. Later when two volunteers showed for a month rates of well over 200, two cases of infection arose in the control population. (58)

> Only 3.9% of Mellanby's patients harboured over 50 mites, with the most heavily infested subject harbouring 511 mites. There are a variety of reasons why patients could have a high mite burden, which will be further discussed. When the mite burden is extraordinarily high, a variant presentation has been described, called crusted or Norwegian scabies. Often such patients harbour tens or even hundreds of thousands of mites and are highly contagious.

11. The unwashed group, however, was understandably more likely to develop infections in their scratched-up skin.

12. Discoverer of the Krebs cycle in biochemistry.

13. Mellanby described his experiments in his classic book *Human Guinea Pigs*, published in 1945, republished in 1973, and again republished posthumously with commentary in 2020. One of the commentaries, written by bioethicist Alastair Campbell, entitled *The 'Untrammeled' Scientist and the 'Normal' Volunteer: Some Reflections*, critically examines the susceptibilities of Mellanby's subjects in the context of their social circumstances, asserting in fact that they were not 'true volunteers'.

14. In the forward to the 2020 edition of *Human Guinea Pigs*, Rob Dunn points out that, 'Subsequent to the time of Mellanby's experiments, ethicists have helped scientists to decide, as a field, that experiments like those Mellanby carried out, in which relatively poor and powerless people volunteer their bodies on behalf of their society, are unethical. But we continue to consider that military recruitment that targets and disproportionately attracts young people with the least power and puts them in harm's way to be, if not unethical, at least relatively unnoteworthy. Why we have decided differently in these two cases is beyond my scope here, but it is a contradiction Mellanby himself is likely to have raised'. (19)

3

The Rash

Cherene

Cherene came to me early in my career complaining of itch, having made a self-diagnosis of scabies. Patients will at times diagnose themselves with all kinds of different maladies, sometimes correct, sometimes not. Any time they can make my job as a diagnostician easier, I regard it as a gift. In her case she had recently travelled to Paris to stay with her daughter and her daughter's boyfriend. Since then both daughter and boyfriend became extremely itchy, and were diagnosed with scabies. Now Cherene was itchy. I knew what to do. Cherene didn't have much of a rash, and no obvious burrows that I noted. However, on close inspection, she had scaling in the web spaces of many of her fingers. Scraping of these areas revealed a pudgy mite when viewed under the microscope. Another case cracked (with patient assistance). Would I have made the diagnosis without the history she provided? Perhaps no, though now that I have many additional years under my clinical belt, every itchy patient gets assessed for the possibility of scabies. 'I knew it', she exclaimed, as I wrote her a prescription for treatment. Her husband, Arthur, who was quietly sitting next to her chimed in, 'should I be treated as well?'

'Are you itchy', I responded? He wasn't. And he had no rash, but was concerned that given the potential for contagiousness, he could contract it. In the course of my dermatology training, I was taught, in scabies, close contacts often acquire the infestation, and should be treated in addition to the index patients. Yes, I learned a lot of stuff in fact. The real trick lies not in learning the material, but rather being able to apply what you have learned in a timely fashion. In this instance, my intuition led me astray. 'You know what Arthur, you look good, and in the same way that you wouldn't need antibiotics if your wife had an ear infection, there is no need for you to treat yourself for scabies', I somewhat dismissively claimed. It almost pains me to pen those words now.

Arthur seemed satisfied with my response at the time, and that time lasted a surprisingly long while. Three months later when he called me back complaining of intense itch, I quickly realized I had made a mistake and backpedalled. 'Uh, please come in, I would like to examine you', I entreated. Sure enough he had burrows and identifiable mites; he had wound up contracting scabies after all. I sheepishly sent a prescription for scabies medication to the pharmacy with a mumbled *mea culpa*: 'I probably should have treated you the first time around.' Arthur was gracious, and I sought atonement by writing a new prescription for his wife, who had no symptoms now, so that they'd both have medication with which they could treat concurrently. I also inquired if there was anyone else in the household that needed to be considered (there wasn't). I had experienced first-hand, one of the prime reasons for failure to control the spread of scabies—treating the patient as if they lived in a bubble. Close contacts should always be simultaneously treated, regardless of whether they are itchy and whether they are officially your patient or not (181).[1]

Dermatology 101: Scabies

So let's put on our dermatologist hats for a minute and review the clinical aspects of scabies. Scabies is an ectoparasite, that is to say an organism that lives, at the expense of humans, on its host's external surface. The pregnant female mite burrows into the uppermost layer of the skin, the epidermis, where it obtains nutrients and lays its eggs, without providing anything in return to its host. It is an infectious disease of the skin, and the skin alone. It does not and cannot invade any other part of the human body. In its quintessential form, it is not hard to recognize. Patients and their family members present with severe itch, often worse at night, with burrows predominantly on the hands, wrists, and often genitals (Figures 3.1 and 3.2).

There is no other skin disease quite like it in this regard. Dermatologist and nondermatologist alike, as well as medical student or other medical professional, can often quickly recognize scabies. Even the lay public can diagnose scabies when the presentation is classic. However, when all the clues are not in place or there is contradictory or misleading information, the picture can be much more confusing. Dr John Stokes, the Director of the Institute of Venereal Disease Control at the University of Pennsylvania and early American dermatologist and venereologist, in 1936, summarized this elegantly with his statement that scabies was 'at once the easiest and the most difficult diagnosis in dermatology'. This still holds true today.

On clinical examination, the finding of burrows is, in medical parlance, 'pathognomonic' for scabies—that is to say a smoking gun, indisputable evidence. As the proverb goes, seeing is believing. Proof of scabies infestation is

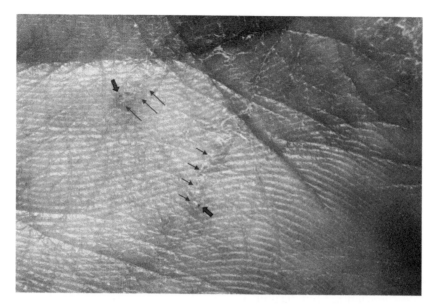

Figure 3.1 Greyish-white meandering lines representing two scabies burrows on palmar skin. These tell-tale lesions of scabies can be easily missed if one does not know what to look for. On the palm, the burrow disrupts the orderly pattern of skin ridges. At the leading edge a triangular speck can be seen by those with excellent eyesight. The thin arrows indicate the location of the burrow, and thick arrows indicate the mite at end of burrow.
Courtesy of Marc Silverstein.

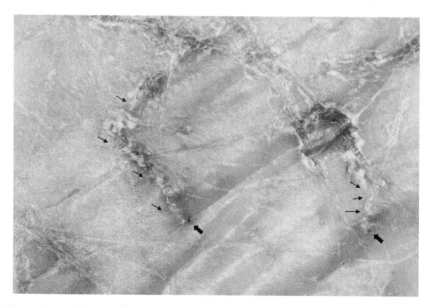

Figure 3.2 Additional burrows. The mite (thick arrows) can be just barely visualized at the leading edge and appears as a triangular dot.
Courtesy of Marc Silverstein.

made by scraping the contents of the burrow onto a glass slide and observing mites, eggs, or faecal pellets (scybala) under the microscope (Figures 3.3–3.5).

When in doubt as to whether burrows are truly present, one can perform the ink test, whereby a felt tipped marker is rubbed over the presumed burrow and then immediately wiped clean with rubbing alcohol. A positive test outlines the burrow with ink that has sunk in and cannot be wiped away. More modern tools used by dermatologists to recognize burrows, include the dermatoscope, a palm-sized handheld surface microscope (Figure 3.6).

Using a dermatoscope, one can even identify a mite at the leading edge of the burrow based on the presence of a small brown triangle, which has been described as the delta-winged jet sign (66) (Figure 3.7).

This corresponds to the pigment present in the mite's head and front legs. The brown pigment at the head of a white burrow has additionally been described as a 'jetliner with its trail' (95), as if it were an airplane soaring high in the sky, with the remainder of the burrow likened to its plume.

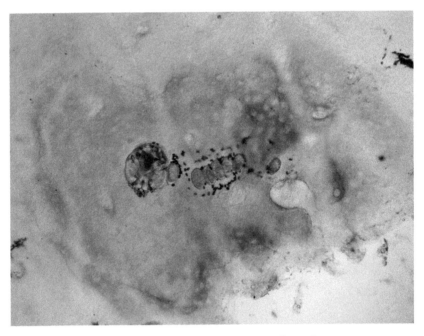

Figure 3.3 Skin scraping demonstrating a mite, several translucent eggs, and numerous smaller dark scattered faecal pellets (scybala). In this scraping technique, the entire burrow has been superficially shaved and placed in mineral oil. Skin scrapings have high specificity but low sensitivity, and a negative scraping does not rule out scabies.
Courtesy of Marc Silverstein.

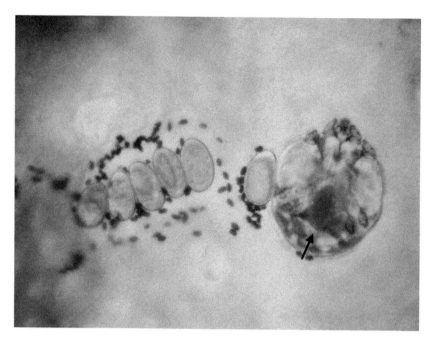

Figure 3.4 Additional magnification of Figure 3.3 reveals that the adult mite body cavity contains an egg which has not let been laid. The darker pigmentation of the mite's head and legs is apparent.

Courtesy of Marc Silverstein.

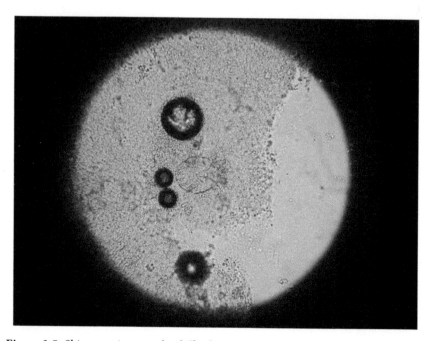

Figure 3.5 Skin scrapings can be difficult to interpret, particularly when the skin is thick. An immature (six-legged) mite lies hidden amongst the scale in between the air bubbles.

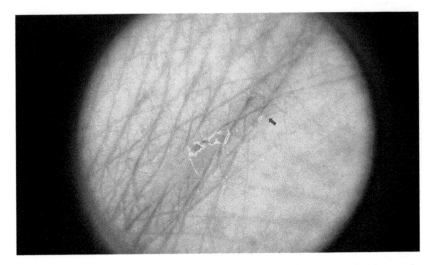

Figure 3.6 View of a burrow through a dermatoscope. The mite can be detected as a minute brown speck at the edge of the burrow (arrow). Ova and faecal pellets (scybala), however, cannot be visualized using dermoscopy.

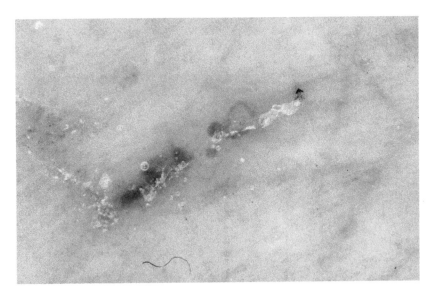

Figure 3.7 Dermoscopy of a burrow, enlarged. At the leading edge of the burrow the mite can be identified by the triangular pigmentation corresponding to its head and legs. Experienced dermoscopists can make a positive diagnosis of scabies based on dermoscopic findings alone. The brown areas of the mite may be harder to detect in darker skinned patients.

Courtesy of Marc Silverstein.

The problem in diagnosis occurs when the tell-tale burrow, is nowhere to be seen. There are many possible reasons for this. One is that the patient may be at an early stage of the disease process before burrowing female mites bearing eggs exist in appreciable numbers. It may be because, as Mellanby observed, some patients harbour very few female mites to begin with. And at times, it may be because the patient's skin has been so heavily scratched that burrows no longer exist or are unrecognizable. In the latter case, patients often wind up with heavily scratched eroded skin which takes on the character of pyoderma or bacterial infection. Treatment with an antibiotic will calm down the skin infection but do little to temper the itch or cure the underlying scabies infection. When burrows cannot be found, the best chance of obtaining proof is by a rather more blind scraping of itchy bumps in the hopes of isolating males, nymphs, or larvae from the so-called larval papules (79, 191). These are small bumps in the skin, often at hair follicles, where immature mites moult as they progress along their developmental cycle.

Interestingly, the typical rash of scabies does not localize to the sites where the burrowing pregnant female chooses to reside (Figures 3.8 and 3.9).

The rash is rather more likely to be seen on the inner arms, around the armpits and waist, and on the inner thighs (both front and back) in a symmetrical fashion. Mellanby postulated that the rash is due to a hypersensitivity, or allergic, reaction that patients developed, possibly at the sites where larval papules most commonly exist. Ferdinand Ritter von Hebra also believed the rash to be a result of hypersensitivity, but thought the distribution was determined by the ease of reach of these sites, and thus directly due to indiscriminate scratching.[2] Irrespective of the underlying reason, the implication is clear. To find a burrow and remove a mite so that one may be definitively able to diagnose scabies, it is not sufficient to examine solely the areas of skin that itch or where there is rash, as very possibly there is no mite to be found at such sites. One must perform a thorough examination with special attention to the areas known to be frequented by the mite. Inspection of the hands, wrists, and the often overlooked genitals is paramount; it is not uncommon for modesty to get in the way. For optimal diagnosis, patients should be unclothed and gowned where they can be examined with good light and a magnifying lens or dermatoscope. Fully clothed or restrictive examination where patients pull back areas of clothing to reveal small surfaces of skin one at a time (known as the 'peek-a-boo' examination) is a barrier to prompt and proper diagnosis.[3]

One of the clinical clues to scabies is that it often is itchier at night-time. Caution must be exercised to prevent jumping to conclusions, however, as many other rashes can also behave this way. As the day winds down, so typically

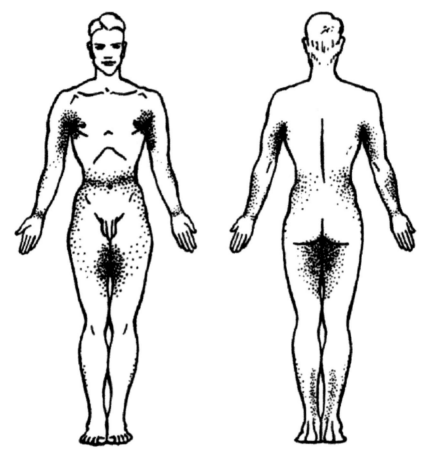

Figure 3.8 Typical distribution of the rash of scabies. Interestingly this does not strictly correspond to the sites where the mite is likely to burrow.

Reproduced from Mellanby, Kenneth. (1972). *Scabies*, 2nd Edition. EW Classey Ltd: Faringdon.

does human activity, and as external stimuli and distractions diminish, all sorts of cutaneous sensations, itch included, have the potential to become magnified. And on the flip side, itching more at night-time is not mandatory for a case to be scabies. Some scabies cases itch equally day and night, and it is not unheard of to see cases that itch more during the daytime. Mellanby's volunteers characterized the itch of scabies as being of three different types: (i) the intermittent itching of almost a biting character which sets in suddenly, (ii) localized skin bump itching, and (iii) diffuse itch sensation in areas where there is little or no sign of inflammation or infestation (8). This last point is particularly worth noting. Such patients having been sensitized to the mite, are often indiscriminately itchy. In less than straightforward cases of scabies, the key to

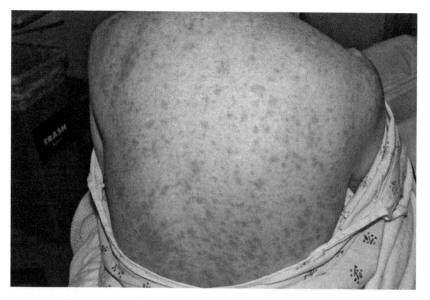

Figure 3.9 The rash of scabies likely represents a hypersensitivity reaction and can be urticarial or hive-like in nature.

making the diagnosis is always to keep it in mind as a possibility. Any and all itchy disorders should at least briefly be considered as possible scabies, whether obvious rash is present or not.

There are several corollaries to Mellanby's observation that sensitization occurs with scabies. For starters, interacting with a known scabies patient does not cause one to develop the immediate sensation of itch. Any display of scratching, discomfort, or anxiety after being around someone with scabies is nothing but the mind playing tricks on itself. Even in the unlikely scenario that one contracted scabies from a patient, itch would not be experienced for many weeks. Second, and clinically more significant, those who don't itch are not necessarily uninfected. Thus at the risk of sounding redundant, it should be reiterated that close contacts of infested patients, whether they are itchy or not, must also be treated. If they aren't, and are infested with scabies in the process of being sensitized, they can serve as a reservoir for the mite and pass it back to the original host—so-called ping-pong transmission. Thus it might come as a surprise that among doctors, including dermatologists, treatment of close contacts is frequently overlooked or conveniently ignored. Last, not unlike in a mosquito bite, the itch of scabies can persist long after the parasite is killed or removed. Such itch can persist up to 6 weeks and can be exceedingly frustrating for patient and physician alike, but is not necessarily a sign of treatment failure.

Sensitization also explains why a previously infested individual who has been cured of scabies will develop symptoms on a much quicker timescale upon subsequent reinfestation. In such persons, inflammation and itching are sensed within a few hours, as their immune system has already been primed. Moreover, because a pre-existing immune response exists, the mite has a harder time spreading. Mellanby found the mite burden to be low in cases of reinfestation, enough so that in some cases vigorous scratching could kill all the mites and essentially cure the disease. Thus it is in fact possible to scratch scabies away.

How exactly is scabies then transferred from one individual to another? Primarily through the fertilized female mite. The most likely scenario is as follows. After hatching, a subset of nymphs will moult and transform into female mites. A female will subsequently burrow slightly into the skin in what might be called a mating chamber. Here she waits to be discovered by a male, upon which mating and fertilization occur. After fertilization, she leaves her mating chamber and wanders on the skin surface until she finds a preferable site to create her egg-laying burrow.[4] Here at this point in the life cycle, the newly impregnated female mite has the opportunity to spread The Itch to others by wandering off onto the skin of another individual. For this to occur however, close, intimate, and usually direct skin-to-skin contact is required. Mellanby summarized this stating, 'transmission is much more often dependent on personal contact, and the more prolonged and intimate the contact the more likely is the parasite to be transmitted' (58).

Once the pregnant female starts her egg-laying burrow, she usually never leaves again. The most common exception would be if she were chased out. The most likely reasons she would be forced out would be due to swelling and inflammation of the skin in and around the burrow (because of host hypersensitivity or even secondary infection) or mechanical dislodgement by the fingernail. In such cases where the pregnant female is forced to leave her burrow, she wanders to a new skin site to create a new home. If she should wander off the skin of her host and onto that of a different individual, she could spread scabies from one individual to another. This represents another potential avenue for transmission. Thus heavily scratched up individuals may represent some of the more infectious cases of scabies, as female mites have been cut loose from their burrows. Ironically, these same heavily scratched up individuals are often the hardest to conclusively diagnose with scabies, as readily detectable intact burrows have been largely scratched away.

And what might be the role of nonfertilized or immature mites in spreading scabies? Presumably these young mites would have a much more difficult time in spreading scabies from one individual to another, as they would be unable to do so without help. For transmission to occur, two developmentally mature mites of the opposite sex would have to independently wander to a new host, meet, up and successfully mate. Or two immature mites would have to wander off, develop into differing sexes, meet, and mate. Based on his experiments, Mellanby thought these both rather unlikely scenarios.[5] And if it were to occur, it would be most common in cases that carry a heavy mite burden, an unlikely (though not impossible) scenario.

For successful transmission of scabies to occur, optimal warmth, humidity, and proximity of individuals is required. These conditions are best satisfied during periods of prolonged intimate contact, such as under bedding. Mellanby humorously alluded to this and insinuated a sexual method of transmission with the double entendre: Scabies is spread 'by picking up a young adult female' (19). And yet, it must be noted that scabies is not exclusively spread through sleeping together in the same bed. Close contact, amongst children or within families is known to be sufficient to spread the disease. Presumably this is due to prolonged proximity of infested individuals next to uninfested individuals.

But what about the spread of scabies through fomites? The term 'fomite' refers to inanimate objects or nonliving things that can carry infection, deriving from the Latin 'fomes', meaning touchwood or tinder (33).[6] For military, as well as public health purposes, fomites have been an object of fascination, study, and overall disagreement, which to some extent continues to the present day.[7]

As with much of our current knowledge, our understanding of fomites rests largely on Mellanby's experiments. As previously discussed, Mellanby found that the average scabietic is infested with only 11 mites. In transmission experiments, Mellanby found that the bedding of patients whose average mite burden ran on the high side (ranging from 20–50), was only responsible for infecting a volunteer with scabies in 4 out of 300 scenarios. Only in patients harbouring more than 200 mites did transmission by fomites become more routine, and even then it was noted only in three out of ten bedding transmission experiments (58). Thus the contagiousness of scabies vis-a-vis inanimate objects seems to be directly linked to the mite burden, or number of mites originally present on the infected host.

Subsequent laboratory studies on the scabies mite have been performed and reveal that under optimal conditions, mites kept away from humans for varying periods of time retain burrowing capability and hence infectivity (9, 11). However under cool and dry conditions, the scabies mite is not a hearty creature. Conditions of high humidity tend to preserve mites the longest. Thus the conclusion that fomites are not responsible for transmission of scabies should be qualified. It holds for locations with dry weather and a temperate climate, such as Europe and North America.[8] In such settings, scabies is a lot more fragile than most people suspect. After being diagnosed and treated, heroic cleaning and decontamination procedures are unnecessary. Simple washing of sheets and towels is a reasonable measure. There is no need to throw away clothing and call an exterminator. In temperate climates, sealing recently worn articles in a plastic bag for 72 hours will suffice to dry up any mites and render them harmless.[9] Other decontamination measures that have been shown to inactivate fomites include freezing at -10 °C for 5 hours, heating at 50 °C for 10 minutes. Scabies contracted in tropical and humid climates, however, behave considerably differently, and here fomites have greater durability and thus are more important in spreading the disease. Recent research suggests that under these circumstances, articles of clothing and bedding need to be isolated for at least 8 days to no longer be infective (158).[10]

In nontropical climates, there is one major exception to the finding that fomites are very unlikely to be responsible for disease transmission. This occurs in the case of crusted or Norwegian scabies (named in tribute to the Norwegian dermatologists Danielssen and Boeck, who first described the condition). In cases of crusted scabies, the mite burden is several orders of magnitude higher than usual. Such patients can harbour hundreds of thousands or even millions of mites. Often immunodeficiency is responsible for this extreme proliferation, and crusted scabies can be seen in cases of HIV, leukaemia, or organ transplantation. Additionally, crusted scabies can occur in those with impaired itch reflexes, such as the demented, the developmentally disabled, those with neurological diseases, as well as the extreme elderly. These cases of Norwegian or crusted scabies are often atypical in their clinical appearance and elude easy diagnosis (Figure 3.10) (204).

Such patients can present with extensive scaling or crusting, and appear to have an extremely uncared for or unwashed appearance.

Their scaly skin, however, teems with scabies organisms, and the flakes of affected individuals can literally harbour thousands of mites (Figures 3.11 and 3.12).

In essence, Norwegian or crusted scabies represents the human analogue of animal mange. Often the multiple and serious medical issues that these patients suffer from make their crusted skin seem like the least of their problems. These cases are clearly much more infectious than others, and can carry a high mortality rate. Because of the huge mite burden, fomites are of greater concern than in garden variety scabies cases, and need to be taken seriously. Careful attention should be paid to cleaning of the immediate environment. Bedding

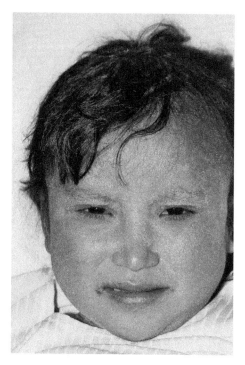

Figure 3.10 Diffuse scaling of the face in a case of chronic crusted scabies. The presentation of crusted scabies is often markedly atypical. Facial involvement in noncrusted scabies would be most unusual, though it occurs with increased incidence in tropical climates.
Courtesy of Jeff Newman.

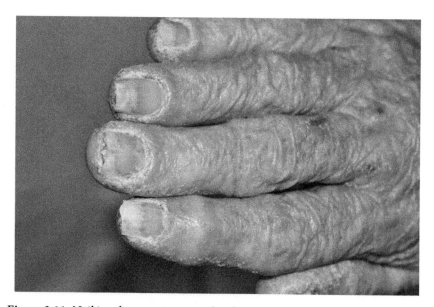

Figure 3.11 Nail involvement in crusted scabies. Scraping of the subungual debris can yield material sufficient for diagnosis in some cases.

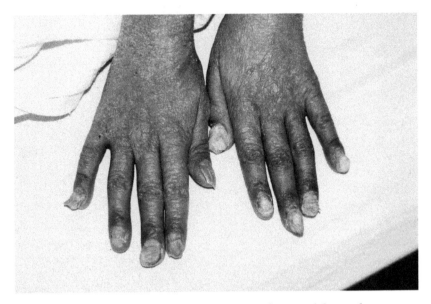

Figure 3.12 When crusted scabies is chronic, significant nail dystrophy can occur.
Courtesy of Jeff Newman.

should be laundered, and furniture carefully cleaned. Floors should be vacuumed, and clothing should either be washed, or tied in plastic bags and left to sit for a prolonged period (12).

Miguel

Miguel, an elderly wheelchair bound gentleman in his 80s who had come to see me, had not had an easy year. Several months earlier, he landed himself in the intensive care unit with a serious infection of the membranes of the brain and spinal canal, called meningitis, which under certain circumstances can be deadly. He managed to recover, and considerably weakened, was sent to a rehabilitation facility to regain strength. With time and physical therapy he was well enough to go home, where unfortunately he fell, leading to bleeding in between the brain and the skull, a condition known as a subdural hematoma, also potentially deadly. Thankfully this condition was promptly diagnosed, and he underwent emergency surgery. Additionally weakened and wheelchair bound, he was sent to a different residential rehabilitation facility where, adding insult to injury, he soon developed a most intense itch on his back. He described it as a kind of torture, as he was too deconditioned to even reach around and scratch himself, though on occasion he feebly attempted using a back scratcher. It kept him up at night, and in spite of all his other medical issues, this was close to problem number one, in his mind. His nursing home physician had snapped a photo of his back and consulted a dermatologist, who decided that something unusual was going on and a more in-depth evaluation would be needed. His doctor had heard I could see him late on a Friday afternoon and hastily arranged medical transportation, no small feat. Through Friday rush hour traffic he travelled clear across the county to come see me, a further indication of his distress. I encountered him sitting in his wheelchair in a cramped exam room, with rumpled hair and full stubble, wearing a medical gown. He appeared to be asleep. I gently introduced myself and he slowly opened his eyes, and gradually leaned forward exposing his back.

Now many an elderly gentleman has an itchy back; it practically comes with the territory. The causes are numerous. Miguel's back, however, was a sight to be seen. It was riddled with dozens of small uniform domed violet bumps. Or were they blisters? At first I couldn't tell and I leaned in wondering if this might be a case of shingles run amok or another unusual viral eruption. But the bumps were firm, and he howled, 'Doc it itches so bad!'

As a dermatologist, there are times when you look at a rash that is distinctive and instantaneously, by dint of training and experience, know what it is. And there are times when you see a rash that is distinctive and think, 'Hmmm, I really should know what that is', which is a troubling realization. This instance fell into the latter category. When that happens, I like to pause, regroup, and collect my thoughts. An itchy rash merits looking around in some more detail, I thought to myself, reverting to a more methodical approach, but also partially stalling. As I glimpsed around, I immediately noted his hands were caked with dry scaling skin, almost resembling powdered dirt. Closer inspection revealed plentiful burrows. 'Fool me once shame on thee, fool me twice shame on me', I thought, as I practically jumped out of my chair. Skin scraping confirmed the now obvious, and Miguel and his wife were given the appropriate treatment.

I made a quick call back to the referring physician who expressed his gratitude but also embarrassment for not making the diagnosis. 'Don't feel bad, it was a pretty atypical case', I reassured him, 'however we'll have to inform the rehab facility management.' He agreed and noted that they would have to invoke their infection control protocol and closely monitor the situation.

Institutional Scabies

Though scabies is not particularly contagious in the general setting, it can be highly contagious under the right circumstances. In institutional settings such as hospitals, skilled nursing facilities, or anywhere individuals reside together in high density, outbreaks of scabies can be seen. Often the scenario involves an initial, or index case, who has unrecognized scabies with a high mite burden, as is seen in Norwegian or crusted scabies (51). Such patients are often misdiagnosed as having psoriasis, eczema, or even dry skin, a rather common finding in the elderly, and can be afflicted with scabies for months or even years while eluding recognition. Often they do not complain of itch (121). Though uncommon, when outbreaks occur in such settings, they can turn into mini epidemics, and quickly become an epidemiological nightmare. Besides lowering morale, and generating bad press, they can be expensive to manage and a challenge to control (131).

When such a scabies patient with a high mite burden also requires frequent and intensive nursing care, the conditions for an explosive situation exist, in which the disease has the potential to spread far and wide. Because itch in scabies develops over many weeks through the gradual process of sensitization, often caregivers and fellow patients become infested without realizing it. Not experiencing itch or any other symptoms, they can thus unknowingly pass scabies on to each other or to close family. Outbreaks of this sort have been thoroughly documented on many occasions.

In one such instance at a community hospital in Southern California, an institutional outbreak of scabies developed which wound up involving over 100 persons (198). An elderly critically ill woman was admitted to the hospital and died 5 days later. Unbeknownst to all, including herself, she was afflicted with scabies. Six days after she died, six members of the nursing unit in the medical tower where she had been cared for came down with itchy bumps on the arms, torso, and thighs.[11] These bumps were nondescript, and the characteristic signs of scabies, burrows, were not present. Only in retrospect was it recognized that these itchy bumps were the earliest manifestation of scabies—representing the larval papules, or sites where immature mites had dug into the skin to further moult. Of the 13 members of the nursing staff who cared for this patient, eventually 9 contracted scabies, an impressive level of contagiousness. Likely the intimate contact required in taking care of this patient—holding her for frequent dressing and linen changes because of incontinence, allowed for mites to directly migrate from the patient's skin to that of the nursing staff. These health care workers thus constituted 'secondary' cases of scabies. Through their close contact with other patients, as well as their own family members, these secondary cases infected a whole new round of people leading to 'tertiary' cases of scabies. All in all 107 persons were affected—66 health care employees, 27 family members of employees, 10 patients, and four family members of patients.

In such outbreaks, the infestation can spread well beyond the immediate nursing and medical staff. At a similar instance at a veterans affairs facility in the early 1990s, a heavily immunosuppressed patient with scabies wound up infecting a host of ancillary staff. These included electrocardiography technicians, phlebotomists, a respiratory therapist, a radiology technician, a patient escort, and a housekeeping worker. The most common site in those infected were the arms and trunk, rather than the hands as might be expected. This may be due to glove wearing and universal handwashing that occurs in such settings (51).

The key to controlling such epidemics is to cast a wide net in determining who should be treated. Some sleuthing is required. Contacts of the infected individual, known, as well as plausible, need to be determined, and should be treated whether they have itchy rash or not (36). Tracking down these individuals and their close contacts is no easy feat, and at times convincing those who feel fine that they need treatment can be difficult. In most instances, topical treatment from neck to toe is suggested. In cases where affected individuals are uncooperative with topical treatment, or in cases where individuals are unable to apply the medication to their entire skin surface, oral treatment, a recent therapeutic development, has been shown to be effective (52).

Johnson

Johnson had newly enrolled in college and was back home for the first time in months for winter break. He had been suffering from increasing itch over the past 6 weeks. He even went to his student health centre where he was prescribed a variety of different steroid creams and anti-itch pills. When they didn't work, his roommates helpfully suggested other potential remedies. He made an appointment to see a doctor, desperate for some kind of relief. He never before suffered from eczema or allergies. Somewhat puzzled, his doctor examined Johnson and only noted a faint pink rash over his upper chest. At that point she decided to send him over to see me.

When I met him, Johnson was sitting on the exam table, fully clothed, holding a bag with a whole medicine chest worth of creams, lotions, and ointments. None of it helped relieve his symptoms for more than half an hour. 'Hmmm, I see', I said inspecting the contents of the bag . . . 'Tell you what, let me step out for a minute and have you fully undress; would you please put on this cloth gown which opens to the back.' Johnson seemed to think that I needed to examine all the potions he had tried and failed, but really what I needed to examine was his entire skin surface. I exited to let him change in private. After a minute, I re-entered and proceeded to examine him from head to toe. His exam was largely unremarkable except for two insect bite-like bumps appearing on the head of the penis and one on the scrotum.

A remarkable clinical pearl that I recall learning as a dermatology resident is that itchy red bumps on the penis are a sign of scabies unless there is a better explanation. For the most part, no other skin condition presents in this fashion. A scraping of the crusts from one of the bumps revealed mite eggs under the microscope. A rush of excitement overcame me, a sensation I still routinely get with a positive scraping (Score!). Johnson was well on his way to having a diagnosis and getting some relief. When I gave him the news, he seemed utterly puzzled that he could have scabies. How could he have gotten it? I had my suspicions. I also suspect he was too modest to disrobe for the initial doctor examining him, thereby hindering their ability to properly diagnose him. I dispensed medication for him and his girlfriend, who was not itchy, and wished him well back at school.

Site Predilection

After many years of practicing, I still find the following fact remarkable: the scabies mite has very clear preferences as to where on the body it elects to burrow. Hypothetically it should be able to burrow anywhere it finds intact epidermis; surprisingly it turns out to be rather picky about the sites where it chooses to reside. At first this can be confusing because, as mentioned, patients afflicted with scabies often seem to be diffusely itchy. This is because the itch of The Itch is immunological in nature and often is sensed all over. In trying to find mites and make a diagnosis of scabies, this can throw the detective off track. Moreover, given Mellanby's surprising findings that there are less than a dozen mites on the average individual, and that half of all patients harbour six mites or less, if one is going to find burrows and successfully diagnose scabies, one better know where to look.

The site predilection of scabies has long been recognized, and its affinity for the male genitalia was described more than 100 years ago (Figures 3.13 and 3.14).[12]

A more complete picture of the body sites where the scabies mite prefers to reside is available, again, courtesy of Mellanby's painstaking work (76). Based on the compilation of his data, analysing the location of nearly ten thousand mites in nearly 1000 individuals, we see that certain body parts are very much favoured over others. Of all the mites he identified, 63.1% resided on the hand or wrist (Figures 3.15–3.20),

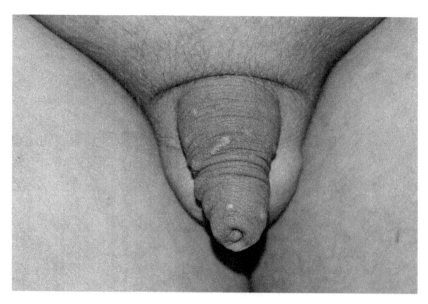

Figure 3.13 Scabies has a predilection for the penis. In this case, a burrow is present.

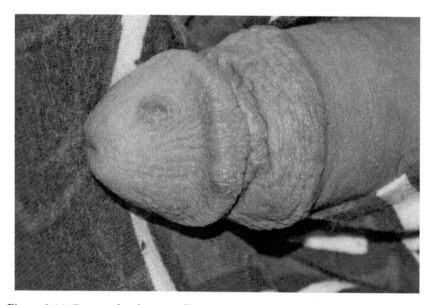

Figure 3.14 Even in the absence of burrows, red itchy bumps or bug bite appearing lesions on the penis are still highly suggestive of scabies. Typically they appear as several in number.

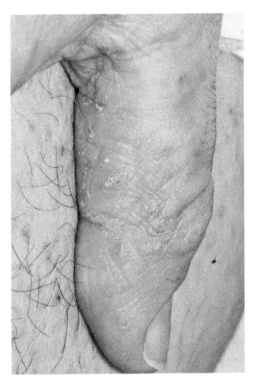

Figure 3.15 Burrows are common on the sides of fingers, where at first glance they may appear as scabs or dead skin.

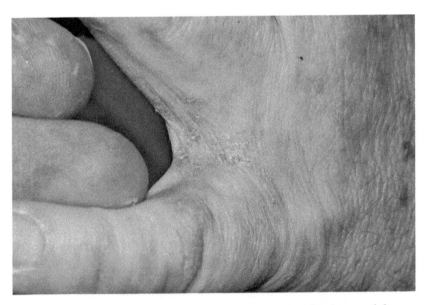

Figure 3.16 Interdigital scaling is a common presentation of scabies, and the interdigital skin is often the first place examined when suspecting scabies. Even if distinct burrows are not clearly identifiable, skin scraping of this area can often still yield mites, ova, or faeces (scybala) under the microscope.

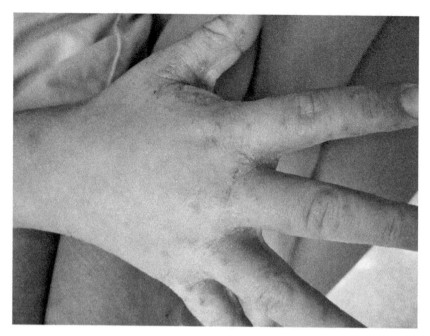

Figure 3.17 Diffuse interdigital redness (erythema), and scaling is present. Epidermal disruption can be present. Blisters or pustules, when seen, are often a sign of secondary infection.

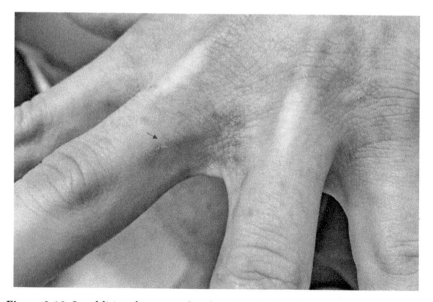

Figure 3.18 In additional to generalized scaling, distinct burrows can be identified (arrow) proximally on the finger.
Courtesy of Patrick McCleskey.

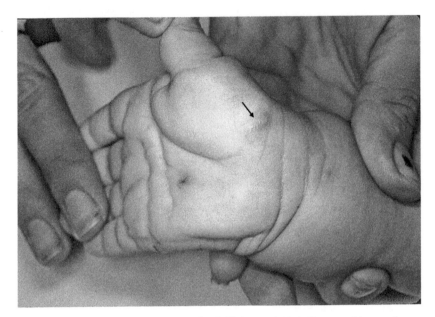

Figure 3.19 A burrow on the wrist of a child (arrow). In infants scabies can be seen on any part of the body, including the face and scalp.
Courtesy of Marc Silverstein.

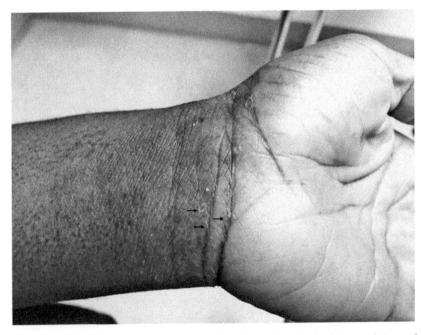

Figure 3.20 Burrows on the wrist of a darker skinned individual (arrows). In such instances, burrows can appear as superficially flaking skin or even air blisters. Burrows in darkly pigmented skin can be more difficult to visualize, and are often seen better on paler areas such as the wrists, fingers, palms, and soles.

10.9% on the elbow (Figures 3.21 and 3.22), 9.2% on the feet and ankle (Figures 3.23 and 3.24), 8.4% on the penis or scrotum, 4.0% on the buttocks, and 2.4% in the axilla (armpit) (Figure 3.25).

Only 1 in 50 mites was found elsewhere. An imaginary circular diagram can be constructed to emphasize these preferred sites starting at the armpit, then passing to the elbow, wrists or fingers, and crotch, and then back, in the reverse order on the other side. Over the years this has been termed the circle of Hebra (Figure 3.26).[13]

In general these are the high-yield areas to examine when searching for burrows. Examination of the fingers and wrists alone, in Mellanby's series, would be sufficient to find a burrow in 85% of cases. And while Mellanby counselled on careful and deliberate examination of all skin surfaces, he noted that from a practical standpoint, when mass screening was required, 90% of scabies cases should be detectable by examination of the hands, wrists, and elbows alone—a great batting average that most any clinician would readily take.

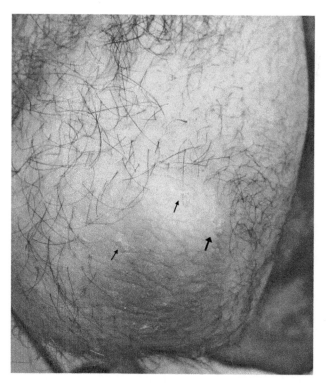

Figure 3.21 Several burrows (arrows) are present on the elbow of a patient with scabies.

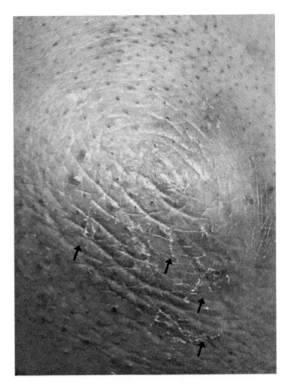

Figure 3.22 Multiple burrows (arrows) are present on this close-up of the elbow.

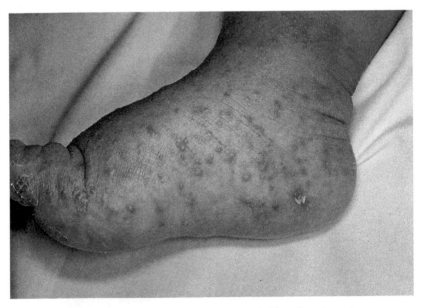

Figure 3.23 Papules and pustules on the feet in a child with scabies. In infants, scabies can appear as small papules and pustules on the hands and feet (acropustular presentation).

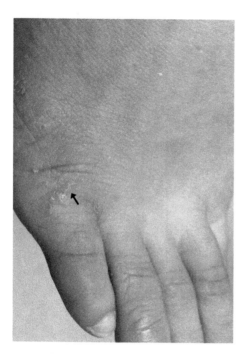

Figure 3.24 A burrow on the foot (arrow) of a patient with scabies. When scabies is suspected and burrows are not readily identified, inspection of the feet is highly recommended.

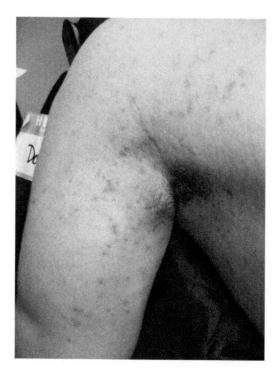

Figure 3.25 Numerous periaxillary papules in a case of scabies.

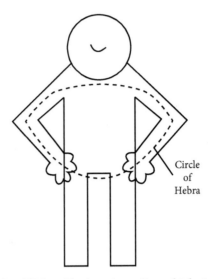

Circle
of
Hebra

Figure 3.26 The circle of Hebra. The imaginary line which circles through many of the main sites of predilection of the scabies mite: axilla, elbow, wrists, fingers, and genitalia. Other common sites include the beltline, buttocks, areola (in women), and feet.

Around the same time as Mellanby, the Danish dermatologist Bjørn Heilesen (1913–2000) independently undertook detailed studies on scabies. Heilesen came from a prominent Danish family with Jewish roots. He studied medicine, graduated from the University of Copenhagen in 1940, and started his scabies research in Copenhagen while under Nazi occupation in 1942. When it became known that the Nazis planned to round up all Danish Jews, he and his family fled to Sweden in October 1943 under the cover of darkness, in a fishing boat, where he was able to relocate and eventually continue his studies on scabies. Heilesen used a dissecting microscope, and often himself as an experimental subject, to study all the steps of the scabies life cycle (Figures 3.27 and 3.28).

He meticulously described 61 controlled experimental infections with scabies, although in a few instances, experiments seemed to get a little out of control—his accounts accordingly make for amusing reading.[14] He published his research in a 1946 booklet entitled *Studies on Acarus Scabiei and Scabies*, which remains an important work to this day for anyone interested in the behaviour of the itch mite.

Heilesen's findings on burrow distribution in scabietic patients are in good agreement with Mellanby's. Heilesen studied the localization of burrows in 123 men and 152 women and found that the vast majority of burrows were found

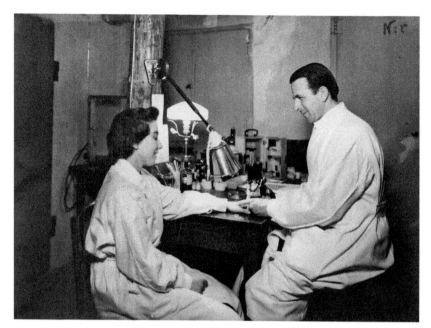

Figure 3.27 Bjørn Heilesen with Berthe-Marie Heilesen, his wife, at his dissecting microscope, working out of a small air-raid shelter room at Saint Göran's sjukhus in Stockholm, April 1945. Many of the scabies experiments that he conducted were performed on himself or his wife.

Courtesy of Simon Heilesen.

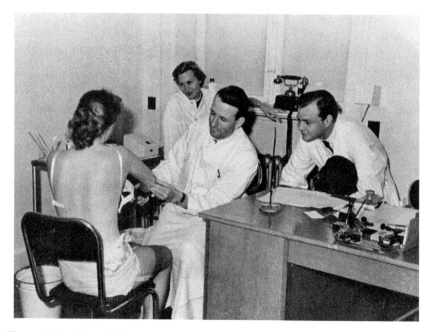

Figure 3.28 Bjørn Heilesen examining patients circa 1952 at Rudolph Berghs Hospital in Copenhagen.

Courtesy of Simon Heilesen.

on the fingers, palms, or wrists. Interestingly, Heilesen found that one third of men harboured mites on their penis or scrotum (8). Nearly 10% of women were noted to have mites on the nipple, whereas in men this was only very rarely observed. Heilesen determined the most common mode of transmissibility was sleeping in a bed with someone else who had scabies.[15]

The site predilection findings of Mellanby and Heilesen, confirmed by subsequent generations of dermatologists, begs the question—why? Why does scabies elect to burrow in these locations? Surprisingly, there is no settled answer to this question, though a variety of theories have been proposed. Heilesen noted that in experimental settings, when mites were moved from one area of skin to another, they often chose to reside in preformed openings made by superficially scratching the skin with a fine needle. This led him to believe that mites preferred topographic features of certain skin sites. He wrote:

> Nobody has yet been able to give a satisfactory explanation of the pronounced tendency of the mites to gather on the sites of election. The investigations of the burrowing of the mite seem, however, to indicate the mites prefer to bore into furrowed or folded skin regions, and have difficulty in burrowing where the skin is quite smooth. Perhaps these observations may to some extent explain why mites only in exceptional cases establish themselves on the back and in the face. (8)

The eminent twentieth-century dermatologist and historian of scabies, Reuben Friedman (1892–1956), postulated that scabies tended to prefer thin areas of skin which were more easily penetrable such as the web spaces of the fingers, the penis, the nipples, and the anterior axillary fold (14). The affinity of scabies for the hands, feet, and elbows, where the skin is thicker than normal, however, would seem to be in direct contradiction to this assertion. von Hebra pointed out that the hands, feet, penis, elbows, and knees, where scabies is readily found, are all sites of pressure, suggesting, along the lines of Heilesen, that this could create natural openings for the mite to burrow in (27).

And what explains the almost universal disdain that the scabies mite seems to possess for the face? In a 1915 article entitled *The Artful Acarus*, New York physician William Cunningham pointed out the lack of general understanding and puzzlement in this regard: 'The exemption of the face and head even in extensive cases in adults, admits of no explanation ... We are forced to the conclusion that the acarus, like its human host, is the victim of idiosyncrasies' (105). It has been suggested that scabies aversion for the face may be due to the increased density of hair follicles found in this area making it hard for the mite to burrow without interruption (29). Heilesen records trying to introduce a mite on the upper part of a volunteer's forehead, noting it had difficulty moving around given the many small hairs present and was only able to successfully burrow when moved to a portion of the forehead where there was only one small hair (8). My own personal theory is that scabies avoids this region because the facial skin is already colonized by a different mite—*Demodex folliculorum*. Sensing this, I suspect scabies avoids this area. Perhaps in the same way that microbes secrete chemicals to fight each other off, the Demodex mite secretes a chemical with antiscabietic properties into the oily follicular secretion known as sebum. Interestingly, scabies is noted to affect the face of infants, whose oil glands are less well-developed and whose hair follicles are less likely to be colonized by Demodex.

Aside from the face, scabies is also seldom seen on the back. For most individuals, the back is a difficult area to reach. Tying these two observations together, it has been suggested that scabies might be spread by the act of scratching oneself (212). According to this theory, either the fingernail spreads scabies from one site to another or the act of scratching causes small furrows which the mite can then use as starting points for further burrowing.

Others have suggested that it is primarily warmth that drives scabies to elect where it prefers to burrow. As the hands are typically kept in close proximity to the sides while sleeping, these areas tend to stay warm, whereas the face, exposed to the air remains cold. Gudden performed an experiment in which he placed a female scabies mite upon the left hand of a man who always slept on the left side, and whose bed clothes were carefully pulled up round his chin. In this scenario a mite was later found on the subject's cheek, presumably having crawled up the arm, and burrowed into the skin of the cheek which 'lay in the warm. The other side of the face remained free from their presence' (39). Along similar lines, the nineteenth-century American dermatologist James White made the interesting observation that those habitually suffering from cold hands and feet rarely were affected by scabies in these parts (84).

Mellanby weighed in with the theory that the hands were the preferred areas of infestation for scabies because they were sites with low potential for inflammation after infestation. He wrote, 'on the hands ... the reaction is often comparatively slight even when the mites are numerous' (76). Possibly this is due to the fact that there is less soft tissue in the hands than other body areas. Other parts of the body with more generous soft tissue would provide an inferior home as they would be more subject to swelling, inflammation, and scratching. The true reasons for why the mite chooses to burrow where it does may incorporate some or all of the explanations discussed in this chapter. The topic continues to fascinate, and further research is required.

Notes

1. The justification for doing so falls under the practice of 'expedited partner therapy' (25, 145, 146). Because prescribing medication for a person with whom you have no professional relationship can be an ethical dilemma, expedited partner therapy has been advocated by the Centers for Disease Control (CDC) under certain circumstances. Originally implemented to help limit the spread of chlamydia and gonorrhoea, it has been suggested that it can be also applied to the treatment of close contacts with scabies. Because treatment with permethrin is quite safe, it seems like a very straightforward case can be made for this practice.

2. von Hebra wrote in his 1868 tome *On Diseases of the Skin*:

   The principal parts occupied by the acarus are the hands, feet, penis, and those spots (such as the elbows, buttocks, and knees) which are subject to pressure. But the excoriations which the patient makes for himself by scratching are found not on these parts, but chiefly on the chest, abdomen, and thighs, over a space which, as a rule, is limited above by a line from one nipple to the other, and below by one from knee to knee. In severe cases of itch the skin of the legs, and that of the forearms and arms, may, indeed, be scratched to some extent; but even then, the face and back invariably remain entirely free from excoriations. Now the only thing to which I can point in explanation of these remarkable facts is the convenience and 'handiness' (das zur Hand-Sein) of the parts which are thus selected by patients with scabies to be scratched for the relief of the itching. It seems as if the patient tormented by the acarus is not (as in the case with persons infected by other epizoa) informed distinctly by his sensations at what spot he is being attacked by his enemy. He feels only a general itching, and therefore scratches most frequently those parts which he can get at with but little trouble, and without much movement of his limbs. (27)

3. In 1893 Philadelphia dermatologist J. Cantrell wrote:

   On inspecting the patient, examine all portions of the body, as you have often seen me do. Do not be satisfied with a peep. Have the patient strip positively as far as the waist. Look first at the hands; examine the sulci between the fingers, the wrists, but do not conclude that the case is not scabies, if you do not find anything upon them, because in Americans, who are, as a general rule, cleanly, we often find that the hands are unaffected. Next the bend of the elbow, the axillae, and parts around the front of the shoulders, the lower part of the abdomen, the lumbar region, and the nipples and breasts of the female, the buttocks and inner parts of the thighs and genitals of the male. If the patient be an infant in arms, look at the face, as this is the portion that comes in contact with the breasts of an affected mother. The feet of infants must also be examined. (134)

4. Mellanby credits the Danish dermatologist Bjørn Heilesen, who will be discussed in future chapters, with many of these observations. More than 40 years after his research on scabies, Mellanby wrote of Heilesen's contributions:

   Heilesen made several interesting observations on the sex life of the mites. He showed that the young female may burrow into the skin, apparently waiting to be found by a wandering male. Copulation then takes place in her burrow. After being fertilized, the female generally emerges on the surface and wanders until she finds a place for a suitable burrow. Copulation probably only takes place once, and renders the female fertile for the rest of her life. (122)

However, not all authors agree on this point. Some suggest that fertilization oc-curs in the egg-laying burrow itself, from which the newly fertilized female never leaves. In addition, some authors believe that immature mite forms rather than the impregnated female are responsible for the transmission of scabies (60). In my opinion, Mellanby's experiments provide compelling evidence that the fertilized female is responsible for the spread of scabies from one individual to another (58).

5. Mellanby noted that it was possible to cure patients harbouring less than 10 female mites by simply physically removing each individual female mite, while leaving the other mites untouched. This suggests that for cases with an average mite burden, young and immature mites are inefficient at procreating and propagating the disease even on the same host, let alone being able to transfer it to another individual (58,76).

6. The use of the term 'fomite' to denote a carrier of contagion was first used by the Italian physician Girolamo Fracastoro, in his 1546 book *De Contagione et Contagiosis Morbis*. In this work, Fracastoro noted that scabies can be transmitted from one individual to another. He is considered one of the founders of the discipline of infectious disease. To protect oneself from catching contagious illness from others, Fracastoro counselled on keeping juniper berries or bark in one's mouth, as well as cleaning one's nostrils with a small sponged soaked with vinegar and rose water. His 1530 poem *Syphilis sive morbus gallicus* relates the story of the shepherd Syphilus, who insults the god Apollo and was thus cursed with the disease now universally known by his name (168). In spite of his advanced views, Fracastoro also believed that scabies could spontaneously generate within the body. Thus Fracastoro, one of the fathers of infectious disease, still believed in the Aristotelian concept of spontaneous generation, which will be discussed in more detail later.

7. Historically, there have been different views on this topic as well. The Italian authors Bonomo and Cestoni in their landmark seventeenth-century description of scabies wrote that scabies was transmissible by fomites. The famous nineteenth-century derma-tologist and scabologist von Hebra believed, on the contrary, that fomites were largely uninvolved in scabies transmission and that disinfection of garments and bedding was a luxury that could be dispensed with. The twentieth-century military physician Captain J.W. Munro, on the other hand, considered fomites to be able to spread scabies. In one instance he reported that clothing from an infected soldier left on the ground for up to 11 days was able to spread scabies to an unaffected volunteer (22). Mellanby, as we have seen, did not think that fomites were a factor in the spread of scabies for the vast ma-jority of cases.

8. It is of course no coincidence that this conclusion is based on research performed in Europe and North America.

9. As recommended by the CDC. Thus in reality, for shutting down exam rooms to do much good, they should also be left closed and out of use for at least 72 hours. The exi-gencies of medical economics dictates this to be more of a ritual lasting several hours than a serious act of infection control.

10. These conclusions are made from experiments using a porcine model of scabies. The human and porcine scabies mite are morphologically indistinguishable from each other. Research on human scabies mites directly is exceedingly difficult to perform be-cause of their limited number on any given infected human host.

11. Here it must be noted that these health care workers developed the symptoms of scabies quicker than would be typically expected for scabies. Exposure to a large number of mites may expedite the development of sensitization.

12. Henry MacCormac in 1917 wrote, 'any system of regimental inspection, for the detection of scabies, must permit of an examination of the whole body and above all the penis' (128).

13. In homage to von Hebra, the illustrious Austrian physician of the nineteenth century who was the first true expert on scabies and one of the fathers of dermatology. His contributions will be expanded on in more detail.

14. In Experiment #18, a young female mite is placed on the wrist of subject BjH (Heilesen himself). The mite stops at a hair follicle and bores down, then turns parallel to the surface of the skin and burrows away from the hair. To limit the spread of the mite, an adhesive plaster bandage is affixed around the wrist. After some additional observations, the experiment is concluded and a local scabicide is applied to terminate the infestation. Except that unbeknownst to Heilesen, the mite was able to escape from the 'ill fitting adhesive plaster'. Approximately 1 week later, while reading, Heilesen develops intense itching of the left elbow, followed by later itching of the buttocks and scrotum. At one point the itching is so intense that he asks the 'catcher of mites' of the clinic to examine him but she [presumably his wife Berthe-Marie Heilesen] only notes a folliculitis. Eventually she also contracts scabies. From this experiment Heilesen concluded that his incubation time for itching was 7 days. He also noted that within 2 weeks, the female mite that escaped was the cause of 15–16 different lesions. The other 60 experiments that Heilesen describes are equally instructive.

15. He drew this conclusion, however, by the questionable methodology of patient interviews. Interestingly, a patient-by-patient analysis of the data shows that men were nearly twice as likely (85% vs 45%) to attribute their contracting scabies to sexual activity, whereas women were as likely to attribute it to sleeping in bed together with a girlfriend as they were to a sexual partner (8). These findings shine light on the social mores of the day.

4

The Mite

Dr N.

I had seen several likely cases of scabies my first year of dermatology residency training. Roughly every other month I would see suspicious case, but my attempts to scrape out and definitively identify the mite would be a failure. Mostly I remember these as exercises in microscope confusion—the lighting, the focus, and what the heck were we supposed to even see? In time we residents learned to master the microscope and spot other pathogens, such as fungi or Demodex mites, but I wasn't making much progress in finding scabies. I seem to remember the same applied for my two coresidents. In cases suspicious for scabies, we would scrape the patient to look for mites, not find any, and then dispense scabies medications anyway on the strength of the clinical presentation. Presumably these patients got better, though sometimes I think back and wonder. The first year of dermatology residency is a busy time packed with lots of new information. Regarding scabies, what I learned that first year was that the mite was pretty clever at hiding—so scabies would be, for the most part, a clinical diagnosis.

I vividly remember the first time I ever saw a verifiable case of scabies. I was in my second year of training, examining an itchy patient. The patient claimed the expected features of intense itch, worse at night, and not responding to the usual remedies; moreover he described having a close friend who was similarly itchy. I thought I knew what to do. I examined his skin, and with a scalpel scraped away at the areas that he claimed were itchiest. Figuring the more skin collected the better, I scraped multiple areas managing to collect a fair amount of scale on a glass slide. I headed over to the microscope, put the glass slide down, added mineral oil and a coverslip, adjusted the eyepiece, and tried to focus. The image I saw consisted of somewhat blurred blobs of skin, highly magnified. I searched around for anything recognizable, without much success. 'Hmmm, again, no luck', I though. I went to present the case to the attending physician Dr N. in the manner that residents do as we go about learning our trade.

Dr N. was a bright young dermatologist that had been recently hired by our academic institution. She had only just very recently completed dermatology residency training herself. I described to her my patient's complaints, and the salient features of his skin exam. 'So what do you think?' she asked me. 'Sounds like scabies', I replied, 'but I got a negative scraping.' 'Really?' Dr N. said peering at me with a sort of surprised but slightly smug look. 'Let's look at what you got', she said and instead of heading to the room to see the patient, we walked over together to the microscope. She sat down and peered into the eyepiece, looking at my sample. She moved the slide around for a bit and then abruptly jumped up exclaiming, 'let's rescrape him.' We headed to see the patient. Dr N. introduced herself, confirmed the history, pulled over the lighted magnifying lens, and brought it to within 6 inches of the patient's hands, where she began methodically examining his hands and fingers, as if she had very limited eyesight. 'There', she said to me, pointing to the area between the patent's thumb and forefinger. 'There what?' I thought. 'Do you see?' she asked. 'That thread of scale on the webspace; it's no more than a few millimeters long. That's where they reside.' Dr N. had just identified a scabies burrow. From her pocket she whipped out a sharp scalpel that she had ready just for this purpose, and in a quick but decisive motion bloodlessly dug out a small amount of scaly skin, without eliciting any pain. She proceeded to deposit the scale on a fresh glass slide. 'If you're lucky sometimes you can find fragments of them under fingernails', she added. We excused ourselves, and headed back to the microscope room, where she sat down to examine her catch, quickly exclaiming: 'Ah ha, there!' Somewhat incredulous, I peered into the eyepiece and in front of my eyes was a pudgy fat butterball, an eight-legged creature that could have been out of a science fiction movie, with scales resembling armour, and bristles running down its legs.

'Wow, so that's how it done', I thought. I had been previously indiscriminately scraping, looking for mites in all the wrong places. On that day, 3 March 2005, commenced my fascination with this parasite formally known as *Sarcoptes scabiei*. Armed with a scalpel, and plenty of practice, I soon evolved to become a quite capable hunter of my own.

Kingdom: Animalia. Phylum: Arthropoda. Class: Arachnida.

So what exactly is this scabies creature? Scabies is a kind of mite, an eight-legged species which belongs to the phylogenetic class of arachnids, which also includes spiders and scorpions.[1] More generally it is an arthropod, an invertebrate with an exoskeleton encompassing a large number of species including six-legged insects as well as crustaceans better known to humans as food in the forms of lobsters, crab, and shrimp, and the like. And most generically, it belongs to the animal kingdom. As Dr Friedman aptly pointed out, scabies is '... as much an animal as is an elephant' (14). Further subdesignation puts it into the subclass acari (derived from Aristotle's *akari*, meaning indivisible), which it inhabits with other minute creatures including ticks. From its flesh cutting properties it acquires it genus name 'Sarcoptes', which is derived from the Greek 'sarx' (flesh) and 'koptein' (to smite or cut). Lastly from the Latin scabere (to scrape or to scratch) we get 'scabiei'. It seems odd, perhaps even creepy, to realize that scabies is an animal that makes its home on human skin. But in fact, that is the case, for which it merits an even more specific designation: *Sarcoptes scabiei var. hominis*. Scabies mites are known to parasitically infest many other mammals (including bats) as well as birds. Typically cross infection from one species to another does not occur or is limited, though experiments demonstrate that it can be possible (57, 65).[2]

The scabies mite is 300–400 microns long (1/75th–1/60th of an inch), with the female being larger than the male, and only just barely distinguishable to the naked eye. Unlike an insect, it is nonsegmented and possesses a stubby head, or capitulum, making it somewhat reminiscent of a miniaturized hedgehog (Figure 4.1).

The scabies mite is flat bellied, with a highly convex or outwardly curved backside, resembling a tortoise in body shape. Its surface is covered with scales, cones, and spines, giving it an armoured appearance of an ankylosaurus minus the tail. The mature mite has eight legs, which are five-jointed. It has two front pairs of legs which terminate in thin walled sacs (or suckers), which help it with balance and skin attachment. The female has two rear pairs of legs which terminate in long bristles. The male differs, however, in that the rear legs are short and terminate instead in thin walled sacs. This feature allows for quick microscopic differentiation between the sexes. The male and female sex organs, on the other hand, are much more difficult to distinguish through conventional microscopy. Pregnant females are readily identified by the presence of an egg occupying a significant portion of their body cavity. By microscopically noting segmentation within the egg, it is possible to determine that a female has been successfully fertilized (Figures 4.2–4.6).

As the lifecycles of the sexes are different, let us first consider the male mite. The role of the male mite is to find and impregnate a female mite. The eminent Scottish dermatologist Alan Lyell wrote, 'the mature males...probably spend a

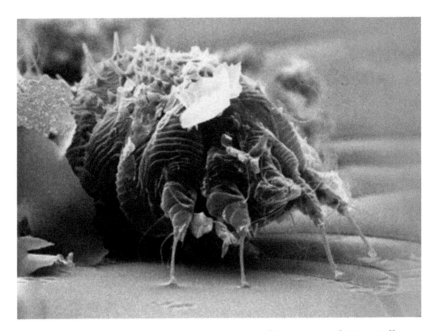

Figure 4.1 Scanning electron microscope image of *Sarcoptes scabiei* partially covered by keratin flakes.
Reproduced with permission from Saari, S. et al. (2019) *Canine Parasites and Parasitic Diseases.* Elsevier.

restless life in search of love' (64). Male mites may tunnel into the skin a short distance for safety, but they do not generate the classic long burrows which are the exclusive purview of the female. Generally they prefer to roam the skin surface in search of a mate, at roughly an inch per minute. When experimentally placed on the neck of volunteers, mites have, on occasion, been recovered from the wrist several hours later, indicating that they can course the surface of human skin in a short period of time (2). Once a female has been located, the male becomes 'agitated, running to and fro and even in circles before suddenly boring into the female burrow' (60). Heilesen studied the mating habits of *Sarcoptes scabiei*, noting that the male had no interest in nymphs, and was exclusively attracted to mature females. By introducing a male mite into the vicinity of a nonpregnant female, he was vividly able to make the following observations (experiment #14):

A lively, uninjured male mite is placed on the skin near the burrow of a non-fertilized adult female. The male keeps quiet for abt. [sic] 1 minute, then starts running about on the skin, apparently without noticing the presence of the

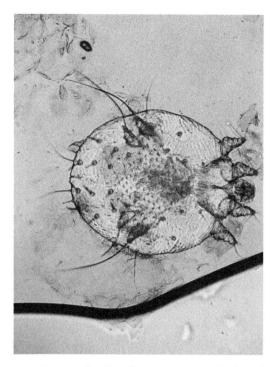

Figure 4.2 Skin scraping reveals a female scabies mite. The front legs terminate in suckers. The long bristles on the posterior legs indicate that this mite is a female. In the male the posterior legs terminate in thin walled sacs. Prominent spines, cones, and thorns are visualized on the body surface.
Courtesy of Patrick McCleskey.

female. At last ... it makes directly for the mouth of the female burrow, which it at once bores into by means of small digging movements. In less than 5 minutes it has disappeared from the surface. It may be just made out through the roof of the burrow that the male rapidly approaches the female, the burrow of which is abt. [sic] twice as long as the animal. 15 minutes after the male was placed on the skin it is seen to be in close contact with the female. (8)

Once in contact, mating takes place. The male mite enters the burrow and approaches the female from behind as if to mount her in the manner observed in many other animals. However just then, surprisingly, while keeping his belly opposed to the female's backside, he proceeds to turn 180 degrees around to face the entrance of burrow. Then, in a manner straight out of the Kama Sutra, he wedges his back against the roof of the burrow while manoeuvring his abdomen against the female's backside such that his horseshoe shaped penis,

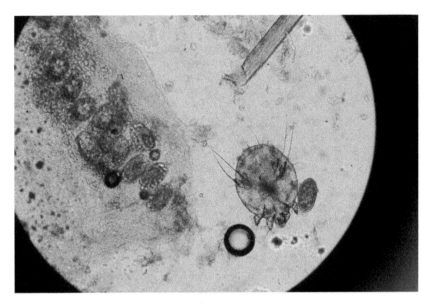

Figure 4.3 A mite adjacent to an egg also showing a burrow with nearly a dozen eggs and plentiful faeces (scybala). Close examination reveals the eggs contain unhatched larva in various stages of development. A hair is seen in the microscopic field which helps to provide a reference of scale.

residing on his underside, comes in contact with the female's reproductive organs (Figure 4.7).

If he is unable to manoeuvre into this position, the male will repeatedly try to reposition himself until he is able to. Heilesen notes that this unusual choreography of copulation is similar to what is observed in the *Tyroglyphus* mite, which is phylogenetically similar to the human scabies mite but instead lives in cheese or flour. The actual act of intercourse, which lasts up to 5 minutes, is extremely rare, though Heilesen reported having seen it on three occasions, though not as up close and graphic as he would have liked: '... how the ejaculation takes place ... it would seem natural to assume that the semen is pressed over into the copulatory organs of the female without the mediation of intromittent spicules, but the question how the transfer of the spermatozoa is effected, must be left open'.

On one of these occasions (experiment #49), Heilesen observed a male and a female mite mating on his skin. In an attempt to capture this act, he applied fixative, anaesthetised his skin with novocaine, and took a biopsy with 'knife and scissors' for more in-depth microscopic examination. Unfortunately, the fixation process was not successful, and no mites were found.

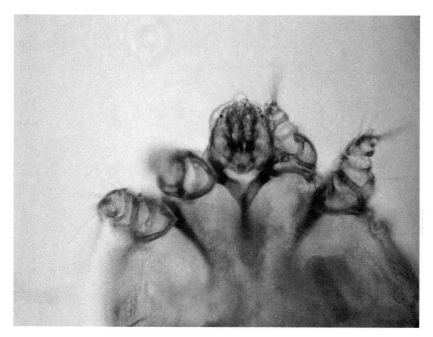

Figure 4.4 Enlargement of the mite's head (capitulum) and forelegs. In this photo, the mandible can be visualized. Heilesen's 1946 publication *Studies on Acarus Scabiei and Scabies* painstakingly lays out scabies anatomy in intricate detail.
Courtesy of Marc Silverstein.

Heilesen furthermore described how after intercourse, the sperm pass from the female's copulatory papillae through the copulatory duct to a spherical sac called the receptabulum seminis, and then through fine tubes to the ovaries, where the egg is fertilized. After approximately 48 hours, the developing egg exits the body through a different pathway than which sperm entered, via the oviduct. The egg then passes out the vaginal birth canal, which Heilesen described as a 'longitudinal slit which rather has the shape of an hourglass, and is bounded by two thick lips lying beneath the birth opening'.

A few days after copulation, the male shrivels up and dies, having fulfilled its role in the scabies lifecycle. The female mite, on the other hand, lives longer. Roughly 6–7 days after mating, she commences egg laying, in the process slowly burrowing her way forward through the epidermis. She lays two to three eggs per day which adhere to the floor of the burrow. Over the course of her reproductive life, the female lays between 10–25 eggs (up to 50 have been noted in one burrow). These eggs hatch in 3 to 4 days, giving rise to an immature larvae that has only three pairs of legs (Figure 4.8).

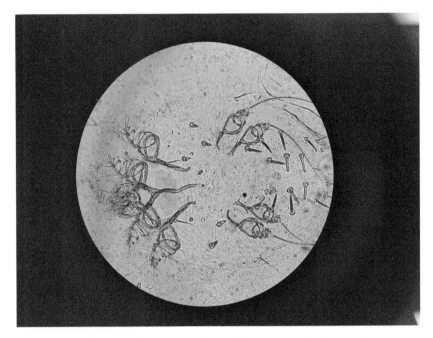

Figure 4.5 Another female mite as evidenced by the long bristles on the posterior legs.

The immature mite proceeds to escape from the burrow likely by boring through the roof to reach the skin surface (60, 104). It transiently roams the skin where it digs in temporarily forming a moulting pouch. Here it morphs into a nymph with four pairs of legs. This often occurs in or around a hair follicle near the burrow from which the larvae emerged. These moulting chambers do not escape the attention of the immune system, and they soon become inflamed, forming small indistinct red bumps also known 'larval papules' (169) (Figures 4.9 and 4.10).

Once in the nymphal form, the immature mite undergoes additional moulting phases before becoming a full-fledged adult. According to conventional dogma, the male and female life cycle are slightly different with female nymphs undergoing an additional moulting stage that males do not. More modern reports dispute this, however, suggesting that male nymphs also moult twice, but that their two nymphal stages (the protonymph and tritonymph) are very similar and difficult to distinguish from one another (59, 62,73). It is only after the nymph moults a second time that its genitals can be observed, and thus determined to be a male of a female.

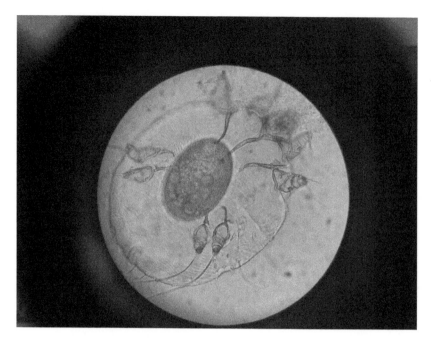

Figure 4.6 A female mite with a large egg in its internal cavity. The egg shows some hints of embryological development.

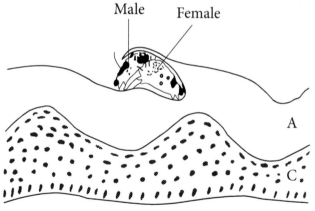

A : Stratum corneum, C : Stratum mucosum.

Figure 4.7 Schematic of scabies mating as determined by Bjørn Heilesen.

Reproduced with permission from Heilesen, Bjorn. (1946). Studies on Acarus Scabiei and Scabies. *Acta Dermato-venereologica*, Supplementum XIV (Volume XXVI).

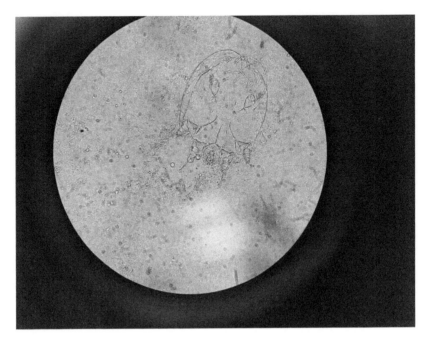

Figure 4.8 An immature mite, possessing only six legs instead of eight.

Given the complexity of the scabies lifecycle with its numerous developmental stages, any individual mite has rather slim odds of successfully developing into an adult. The human immune system and fingernail are, as we have discussed, its prime enemies, but immature mites are inherently not hearty creatures. Heilesen noted that, 'the larva has not the same capability as the female mite to adhere to the skin, a breath of wind in the laboratory could sweep it away'. Mellanby determined that in most scabies infected individuals the number of mites present on the body surface peaks between day 80 and 115, after which it begins to decline (58). During this period, if all the eggs laid were to hatch and successfully develop into adult forms, nearly three quarters of a million mites would overwhelm the human host. This is essentially what is seen in Norwegian or crusted scabies, where immune and neurologic defects are largely responsible for the mite population explosion which goes unchecked. In ordinary cases of scabies, however, the mite burden is usually in the tens not the tens of thousands. The odds are very heavily stacked against any given larvae successfully maturing and surviving to adulthood.

For the vast majority of her life, the adult female scabies mite resides in a burrow that she creates in the keratin-rich outermost layer of skin cells called the stratum corneum (Figure 4.11).

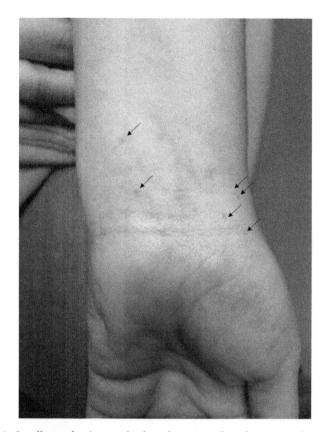

Figure 4.9 Small papules (arrows) where larva moult to form nymphs, or the so-called larval papules, are present on this patient's wrist. When burrows are not readily recognizable, larval papules are the next highest yield areas to scrape in searching for evidence of scabies infestation.

This layer is comprised of decomposing skin cells known as keratinocytes. These keratinocytes are born deep in the skin at the junction of the epidermis and dermis, and slowly rise to the surface, where they thin out, lose their cellular subcomponents, and eventually slough off, a process taking approximately 14 days from start to finish. The female burrows forward through the stratum corneum, laying her eggs and haphazardly depositing her faecal waste (Figure 4.12).

At the very front-most part of the burrow she dips her head into the slightly deeper layer of skin called the stratum granulosum. From here, where keratinocytes are still nucleated and alive, she obtains nourishment and moisture (101). Her burrowing is executed in an exquisitely choreographed fashion pitting the

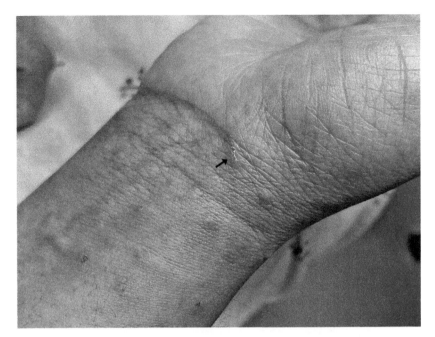

Figure 4.10 Larval papules, many excoriated, are noted on the ventral wrist. A proper burrow (arrow) is also visualized.

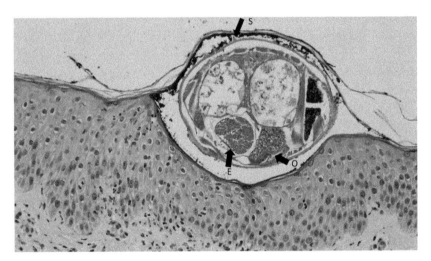

Figure 4.11 A photomicrograph of a haematoxylin and eosin stained section taken from a skin biopsy. The mite is located in the stratum corneum, the most superficial layer of the epidermis. Small spines (S) on the surface of the mite can be visualized. The kidney bean–shaped subcellular structure is an egg (E) in development; immediately adjacent to this is a portion of the ovary (O) showing oocytes with prominent basophilic nuclei which will develop into ova.
Courtesy of Joanne Sung.

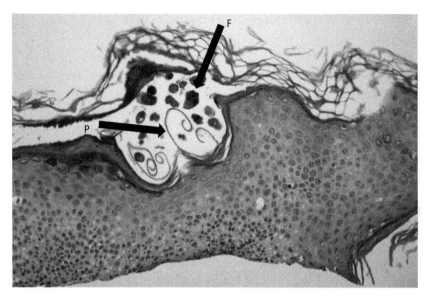

Figure 4.12 A photomicrograph of a haematoxylin and eosin stained section taken from a skin biopsy. While no mite is visualized, a diagnosis of scabies can be made from the brown amorphous globules which are scabies faeces (F) also called scybala. The curled pink structures are known as pigtails (P), and are remnants of scabies eggshells or casings.
Courtesy of Max Fung.

timing of her lifecycle against the skin's shedding and regenerative cycle. As skin sloughing proceeds, she continues to burrow forward (and down) so as to not be sloughed off herself. Her eggs hatch in 3–4 days such that her larva can escape as well.

Female burrowing activity was once thought to be exclusively mechanical in origin. By biting her way forward with her jaws and using her spined legs to hook and propel herself onward, the female mite was depicted as using sheer force to burrow through the epidermis (8, 60). Munro's vivid description from nearly a century ago is that of a mite digging into the skin:

> The ovigerous female . . . fixes on to the skin by the suckers on her anterior legs and, propping her body up with bristles on her posterior legs, assumes an almost perpendicular position and commences cutting into the skin. She very soon bores in, being completely concealed in as short a period as two and a half minutes. (22)

Heilesen describes a similar process (experiment #42):

On the l. wrist an adult lively female is placed near the tail of a tattoo-mark of a snake. The mite immediately begins to bore in, and in doing so is in a position which is favorable for the observation of the burrowing. The animal bored the capitulum into the side of a furrow in the skin, moving it alternately towards the r. and the l. medial foreleg. It was actually seen how a small slit was made in the epidermis and a small scale was partly detached ... Continuing the burrowing the animal bores now to the right, now to the left, in this way so to speak 'elbowing' its way on, into and downwards in the epidermis.

More recent studies, including scanning electron microscopy (103) of the scabies mite in its burrow, suggest that the act of burrowing is as much chemical in nature as it is mechanical (9, 31, 47, 104). From its large salivary glands, the scabies mite secretes enzymes that help dissolve the stratum corneum, allowing it to sink in. Small remnants of skin cells have been found in the gut of scabies as well as in its faecal pellets. Thus the mite actually ingests portions of the host skin as she burrows forward (104). The mechanism of burrowing is likely a complex choreography of both enzymatic and mechanical steps.

Once burrowed in, the female mite begins egg laying. Sooner or later, the mite elicits an unwelcome host inflammatory response. To evade this, as well as seek new sources of nutrition, she burrows forward at the rate of several millimetres per day. The immune response is directed to the segment of the burrow that has been enzymatically altered by the scabies mite, and where its saliva and faecal remains are found. But by this time, she has burrowed ever so slightly forward and in this fashion, she is constantly on the move to elude the immune response, staying a few millimetres ahead of it. The immune response consists of a white blood cell exudate, which manifests as swelling, and at times a small blister or pustule. Historical texts are replete with references to the blisters or pustules seen in scabies.[3] In my experience, blistering associated with burrows is unusual and, when present, is apt to be scratched into a scab or dried out into a crust. It is likely that in the prior era of reduced cleanliness and less attention to hygiene, blistering associated with the scabies burrow was a more common feature. So much so that physicians of the day, many who had no concept that a burrow let alone a mite even existed, would use the presence of such blisters in the context of severe itch as a surrogate finding to help them make the diagnosis of scabies.

The fact that the mite and the vesicle are located at different places along the burrow, separated by no more than a centimetre at most, has wound up being a great source of confusion for those trying to discover the true cause of The Itch (17) (Figure 4.13).

It literally and figuratively has allowed the scabies mite to stay one step ahead of those trying to catch it. For here in the blister fluid, physicians and scientists have searched for scabies, a fruitless task as it not where it resides. And when they were unable to find the mite that others had described to cause scabies in the blister fluid, their conclusion was that no such mite existed. Ironically it was not physicians but rather lay healers who figured out that to find the mite one needed to look at the tip of the burrow and not in the adjacent blister fluid. The key to proving that scabies was due to a mite, the ability to reliably reproduce it time and time again, lay in realizing that the often-observed blister is a

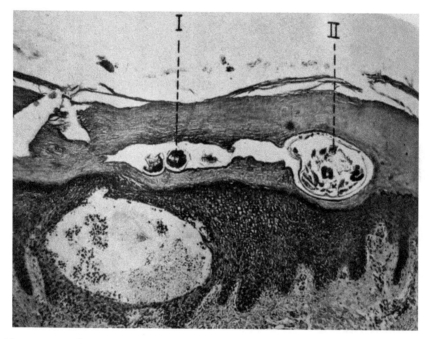

Figure 4.13 Photomicrograph of a haematoxylin and eosin stained section taken from a skin biopsy. The mite (labelled II) has clearly advanced past the area of cutaneous inflammatory cells. The scabies mites constantly burrows forward to avoid the host immune response, and is not found at the site of the skin pustule (large oval within epidermis, below label I). Rather it resides at the most forward tip of the burrow. Being unable to find the mite in the pustule led many early investigators to conclude that mites were not present in scabies, thereby delaying our understanding of this disease by several hundred years.

Reproduced with permission from Heilesen, Bjørn. (1946). Studies on Acarus Scabiei and Scabies. *Acta Dermato-venereologica*, Supplementum XIV (Volume XXVI).

secondary phenomenon. The itch mite is to be found at the leading edge of the burrow. Today this simple fact seems rather obvious. However, as we shall see, it did not gain scientific currency until the early nineteenth century.

Up until very recently, research on scabies had been performed almost exclusively in temperate or dry climate regions. Only in the last decades has it come to our attention that the life cycle and clinical characteristics of scabies in tropical or humid climates assumes a rather different character. In tropical settings, the mite often does not burrow into the skin, as the environmental warmth and humidity afforded make this unnecessary. Thus in tropical climates, classic burrows are often not seen (4, 71, 120). Instead the female mite roams the surface residing in ridges, possibly at the base of hairs, or in other favourable topography, or she digs into to the skin very superficially. In such instances, individual lesions are described as small bumps (papules) or pustules (7, 34). This can make scabies a challenge to diagnose in this setting. In addition, under humid conditions, mites are more hearty and less quick to desiccate. It has been shown that high levels of humidity prolong the survival of canine mites and their ability to reburrow into their host at all but the hottest temperatures (9, 72, 132). If these findings correlate to human mites as well, it would seem that fomites in tropical settings should have greater potential infectivity.

Tropical scabies diverges from classical scabies in several other aspects. For reasons not understood, the distribution of lesions in tropical climates is unique, with a greater likelihood of involving the skin of the neck, face, scalp, and skin folds behind the ears (31, 37). With the exception of infants, these are not areas frequented by temperate climate scabies. Additionally, in tropical climate scabies, those affected are more likely to develop bacterial infections in their scabies infested skin, which as will be later described, can lead to devastating consequences, particularly in children. Because of such differences, tropical climate scabies should be considered a distinctive and major variant of scabies, and it deserves special mention in dermatology texts and other educational materials.[4]

Notes

1. Many different types of mites can be found in nature. They are found in fresh, brackish, and salt water as well as on land. They can live on a variety of objects including animals, grains, straw, dust, dried fruits, and other foodstuffs. The flour mite, *Acarus siro*, can impart a pungent order, described as 'mintiness', to flour and render it unsuitable for eating (173). The cheese mite, *Tyrophagus casei*, on the other hand, imparts unique flavours and is a natural part of some cheesemaking processes.

2. One of the best reviews of current knowledge regarding scabies biology is that of Arlian and Morgan (132).

3. Munro, in his scholarly 1919 review of scabies, writes:

> [...] the vesicles [blisters] are small, about the size of a grain of barley. They are the result of irritation caused by the acarus secreting an acrid fluid, and while they invariably denote than an acarus is present in their neighborhood they do not always indicate the precise position of the mite. They may occur some distance from the egg burrow. On their being opened a serous fluid exudes from them. They are often ruptured by the scratching of the patient, and, on healing, form minute crusts. (22)

4. Perhaps the best account of scabies, in general, and specifically tropical scabies in current didactic material is found in Tyring, Lupi, and Hengge's *Tropical Dermatology* (120).

5

Epidemiology

Scabies and Its Periodicity: The 7-year Itch?

An odd and rather interesting feature of scabies is that it has been noted to occur in periodic or cyclical outbreaks. Mellanby wrote, 'all records from both recent and medieval literature suggest that scabies has always been a disease which has come in waves'. Many patterns have been proposed though none has been clearly established. The twentieth century has reportedly experienced major outbreaks of scabies from the years 1919–1925, 1936–1949, and 1964–1979, leading to the hypothesis that it has a defined periodicity.

If indeed scabies epidemics occur in a cyclical fashion, the underlying rationale for this may be attributable to the waxing and waning of population-wide immunity, a concept known as 'herd immunity'. The scenario might be expected to proceed as follows: during times when exposure to scabies is rare, overall immunity to scabies in the general population (herd) would be expected to be low. If a mite should gain access to such a population of individuals, it would be able to spread extensively. Its spread would be aided by the rather long incubation period scabies demonstrates in the immunologically naive host, in effect giving it a head start to propagate widely before causing symptoms and becoming recognized. Meanwhile, not having been prevalent for some time, the medical community would be slow to recognize the outbreak.[1] All of these elements combined would lead to potentially explosive dissemination. In a relatively short period of time, scabies would become widespread. At the point where it reached a pandemic level, the nature of the outbreak would change. The clinical presentation of scabies would be more readily recognized. Infected individuals would get treated, and precautions would become more routine. In the case of re-exposure, previously treated individuals would maintain immunological memory, thereby mounting an immune response readily, making reinfection more difficult. Eventually the general population would come to attain a certain level of immunity to scabies, thereby limiting the ability of it to spread further. As it spread less, it would become rarer, and with time, fewer and fewer individuals would become exposed. Slowly scabies-specific immunity, as well as general recognition of the condition would diminish, at which point the cycle would repeat (30).

Of course, much remains to be understood in this hypothetical scenario. Whether there are features of the mite lifecycle that inherently lead to cyclic outbreaks or whether periodicity is related to external factors, such as war, displacement of human populations, and the relaxation of sexual mores, remains a matter of debate. It has also been suggested that the concept that scabies has a fixed periodicity is an oversimplification of the data (31, 74, 120). Part of the difficulty in comprehensively understanding the epidemiology of scabies is that, unlike many other contagious illnesses, scabies is not a mandatorily reportable disease in most jurisdictions.[2] This makes it difficult to track and study. Moreover, it has been noted that in some areas scabies is endemic without fluctuation in incidence whatsoever (38, 62).

And if scabies has a periodicity of upwards of 20 years, what then should be made of its colloquial moniker 'the seven-year itch'? Exactly where does this term come from?[3] Some have suggested that this refers to its prolonged course when untreated or improperly treated (7). Others have suggested the term originates from the Napoleonic Wars (31). During this series of conflicts at the beginning of the nineteenth century, scabies was epidemic with upwards of 400,000 French soldiers afflicted (Figure 5.1).[4] Cases of scabies under wartime conditions of the day were particularly prone to serious secondary infection and were one of the prime causes of casualty in the military (60).[5]

By any objective reality, the true attribution of the term 'seven-year itch' remains obscure, and I have yet to pinpoint its origin.[6] My own theory is that the term derives from the impact of scabies during the Seven Years War, also known as the third Silesian War of 1756–1763. In this conflict, Prussia defeated Austro-Hungarian forces in Central Europe, thereby elevating itself to the status of a major European power. In the fighting, multitudes were reportedly ravished by scabies. The German military surgeon Dr Klehmet described the scene more than a century ago, writing:

> During the Seven Year's War, itch was one of the commonest and most serious diseases; in many cases half the men of a regiment were in hospital at one time for this complaint. Baldinger, a surgeon in Frederick the Great's army, has recorded the fact that he often saw soldiers whose whole body was covered with masses of greenish moss-like scabs, the result of itch. The disease was ascribed to foul emanations in the overcrowded hospitals, to the debilitated condition of the men, and to want of personal cleanliness and deficient

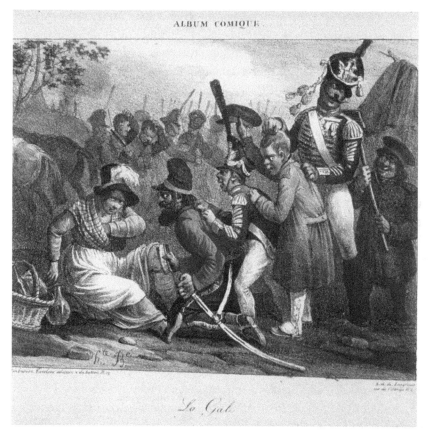

Figure 5.1 A line of unusual characters scratch each other in Le Gale painted by Hippolyte Bellangé in 1823, more than a decade before Renucci's dramatic demonstration of the scabies mite.

perspiration. Everyone in the army from highest to lowest was sooner or later attacked by this disease. Owing to the universal custom of billeting troops on the inhabitants, the civil population also suffered severely. Intimate contact with horses was supposed to be a certain preventive, as it was found that cavalry soldiers did not suffer to anything like the same extent as infantry men; the real explanation probably was that the cavalry were billeted in farms and not placed in barracks. (83)

The German physician and scabies pioneer Johann Ernst Wichmann (1740–1802) in 1786 wrote a contemporaneous account in which he also related that scabies was widespread in the Seven Year's War:

Every physician familiar with military hospitals knows that virtually no patient in these hospitals is safe from scabies. An incident which occurred in the Seven Year's War shows that not even the greatest Commander-in-Chief [Frederick the Great] is any more safe from infection with this disease than is a common musketeer should the former accept a letter, or anything at all, from the latter's scabetic hands.

Memory of the scabies outbreak in the Seven Year's War led the Prussian army to undertake precautions in the subsequent Napoleonic Wars nearly 50 years later. After the fighting had concluded, Prussian troops were required to undergo a medical exam and be certified scabies-free before being allowed to return home (14). It is but speculation, but perhaps what was once known as the itch of the 'Seven Year's War' became abbreviated and simply known as 'the seven-year itch'.

Craig

Craig presented to the Residents' clinic on an autumn day in my third and final year of residency. Residents' clinic was much like it sounds—a clinic run by the residents, dermatologists-in-training, where, over the course of 3 years, we would see and follow up on our very own patients. According to our level of experience, we would seek out help in making diagnoses and establishing treatment plans from more senior physicians. As we gained experience, we transitioned to taking care of these patients on our own, with less outside help as time went by. In short, Residents' clinic was a way of letting those of us in training run the show, under supervision.

Craig was a heavy-set individual with extremely thick glasses. He was accompanied by his sister and mother. Craig had Down's syndrome, also known as trisomy 21, which imparted mild intellectual disability. He was very pleasant, even charming, 'Hi I'm Craig, we have the same name', he introduced himself. After some pleasantries, his sister related the details of his skin problem. Craig had been suffering from an itchy rash for months now, which was showing no sign of going away. Apparently the usual retinue of salves and steroid creams had not helped.

I sat down next to Craig, and repositioned his gown to examine him. Inspection revealed pink dry skin with plentiful scratch marks all over his torso. Notably, he had very prominent crusts and scaling on the instep of both feet. Suspecting that he might have a bad case of athlete's foot, I explained to him that I wanted to take a small scraping for microscopic examination. 'OK Craig', he replied.

A quick scraping and trip to the microscope did not result in what I had expected. When I looked in the eyepiece, instead of seeing branched stringy filaments of fungi, several pudgy mites with thick stubby legs containing long bristles jumped out at me. 'Wow', I thought to myself, 'fooled'. Here was a case of scabies, not foot fungus.

I called my fellow residents over, and suggested they introduce themselves to Craig and ask for permission to examine him. While they were doing this, I presented Craig's case to one of the supervising physicians, a grey-haired dermatologist who over his long career had seen it all. He peered in the microscope, and nodded with a slight smile. Slowly the residents who had gone in to see Craig came out and I directed them over to the microscope as well. A series of ahas! ensued.

I went back in to explain to Craig and his family that he had scabies, and I then prescribed topicals medication to all three of them to use concurrently. 'Craig, I suspect in a few weeks you will be feeling much better', I reassured him. To which he replied, 'Thank you Craig, I'm so happy you are my doctor.'

Those at Risk

So who gets scabies anyway? In fact, all humans can get scabies. The minimum requirement is to have skin. In his 1947 book, *The Story of Scabies*, Dr Friedman summed up this sentiment, writing, 'The *Acarus scabiei* [*Sarcoptes scabiei*] is notorious for its lack of respect for person, age, sex, or race. Whether it is in the epidermis of an emperor or a slave, a centenarian or a nursling, it makes itself perfectly at home with undiscriminating impudence and equal obnoxiousness.'

Having duly noted that just about anyone can contract scabies (183), it must be pointed out that various groups of populations tend to be at higher risk. For starters, the most immediate and primitive defence against scabies is the fingernail. Those who, for one reason or other, cannot or do not scratch tend to be at increased risk for contracting scabies. This includes the very young, the very old, the developmentally delayed, the institutionalized, or those with diminished immune responsiveness.

Both ends of the human lifespan are particularly susceptible to scabies. Infants are prone to developing scabies because of the close physical contact they have with their caregivers, as well as their inability to communicate verbally. Often, scabies in infancy is not easily recognizable, with the main manifestations being irritability and poor feeding (78). The elderly are also particularly prone to scabies. Dementia is a documented risk factor for scabies (121). Other neurological or psychological problems that mask itch, seen with increased incidence in the geriatric population, can allow scabies to go unchecked (121). When scabies fails to attract the attention of the host it can easily run rampant. As discussed, the clustering of elderly in communal settings such as retirement homes can additionally lead to the spread of scabies where outbreaks can be explosive, quickly turning into mini-epidemics.

Immunosuppressed patients are another group that tend to be susceptible to scabies. A weakened or deficient immune system can lead to an inability to mount an effective immune response to the mite. This group includes those who have HIV/AIDS, those who take immune suppressing medications, those who suffer from various forms of cancer, and those who for genetic reasons mount an ineffective immunological response.[7]

Close physical contact is another risk factor for contracting scabies. This is particularly seen in urban or other areas of high population density (69), or under conditions where human beings tend to huddle together, such as during the winter.[8] von Hebra in 1860s Vienna had noted scabies to be seven times more likely in men than in women, which he attributed to the custom where male apprentices often slept together in the same bed. 'In this city [Vienna] scabies is most frequent in those trades in which the apprentices sleep two in a bed. The shoemakers furnish forty to fifty per cent, the tailors twenty to thirty per cent of all cases' (14).

In resource-poor countries where children live in crowded conditions, children often spread scabies amongst themselves by nonsexual contact such as hand holding, cuddling, or care-giving. In some instances, children can then proceed to introduce scabies to their entire family. Socioeconomic risk factors for scabies are difficult to determine in resource-poor areas. In many such areas, the resources for diagnosis are limited, and a diagnosis often has to be made based solely on clinical criteria, such as the presence of itch worsened at night, noted in multiple household members. The general assessment is that poverty promotes scabies (186), though this may be more a function of crowded quarters. One specific study from Bangladesh in the mid-1980s suggested that risk factors for scabies included not owning the house one lived in, as well as lack of electricity (174).

Sexual contact also predisposes one to scabies, though scabies is really more a disorder of physical closeness rather than actual sexual contact in itself.

Prolonged bed-sharing allows mites to migrate from one person's skin to another. Accordingly, the diagnosis of scabies is suggested when sexual partners, or multiple family members simultaneously complain of itch. Mellanby poked fun at the sexual method of transmission recalling the following ditty (19):

Recondite research on *Sarcoptes*
Has revealed that infections begin
On leave with your wives or your children
Or when you are living in sin,
Except in the case of the clergy
Who accomplish remarkable feats
And catch scabies and crabs
From door handles and cabs
And from blankets and lavatory seats.

It is currently estimated that between 130 and 230 million individuals worldwide suffer from scabies (91, 93), with a particularly high concentration in the tropical zones of East Asia, Southeast Asia, Oceania, Latin America, and South Asia (213). Aside from the maddening itch and severe discomfort it causes, scabies also confers increased risk of bacterial infection, which can lead to serious consequences, especially where access to medical assistance is limited (202). The scabies mite tracks bacteria as it burrows through the skin, both of which can be spread by scratching.[9] The proliferation of *Staphylococcus* and *Streptococcus* bacteria, can lead to a honey-coloured crusting of the skin, an infectious complication known as impetigo. Impetigo can mask the diagnosis of scabies; however, more ominously, it can trigger a cascade of events leading to kidney damage. This occurs when the body's immune response to the bacteria leads to inadvertent inflammation of the kidney, a process known as glomerulonephritis. Scabies related poststreptococcal glomerulonephritis amongst children is a leading cause of long-term kidney disease in developing tropical nations (28, 100). There is also some evidence to suggest that through a similar mechanism, scabies related impetigo could be a trigger for the development of rheumatic heart disease (100). Thus scabies, and scabies related impetigo, especially in developing tropical countries is not strictly an itchy nuisance—it can cause considerable morbidity and long-term health problems. Recognizing this, the World Health Organization has recently officially designated scabies as a neglected tropical disease, highlighting the need for additional research and resources (5, 99, 199, 203, 213).

Conditions of Misery

Like other infectious diseases, scabies can run rampant under conditions of crowding, poverty, poor hygiene, and malnutrition. Outbreaks in refugee camps (115, 130), prisoner-of-war camps (118), and 'immigrant detention facilities' have been documented, and occur to this day,[10] compounding the general misery already present in such situations. These localized epidemics among very vulnerable human beings already in crisis, are a pointed reminder of the failings of humanity.

La Migra
Bert Johansson MD, pediatrician El Paso, Texas

Native people have been using the natural breaks in the mountains and rivers that cross our continent to traverse north and south for more than a millennium. More recently, many people have crossed the Southern Border in search of work and a better life in the United States. In the past decade, there has been a change in the demographics of those crossing the border. We have seen a transition from predominantly Mexican males headed North for work, to more recently, migrants from Honduras, El Salvador and Guatemala, many families, mostly women and children headed north for el Milagro del Norte, the American Dream. They are fleeing oppressive governments, wars of genocide (many are native people) and vicious drug gangs that operate with impunity in their homelands. Tens of thousands have fled north in the past year alone, navigating unforgiving terrain and hostile people; if they choose an eastern trail north they must travel through Tamaulipas where they endure centuries old tribal hatred or if they take a more western trail they must pass through Sinaloa and contend with the powerful drug cartels and their sicarios (hitmen or assassins). If they make it to the US-Mexico border they encounter immigration and law enforcement officials and a currently unwelcoming political climate.

When Border Patrol notified us that 200 more Central American asylum seekers, 'most of them children', were being released into our shelter system, we mobilized. Since 2014 we have responded and grown accustomed to, but are not inured to the periodic release of migrants. This night was no different, except that the children being released had been held for 'a prolonged period' in a facility that had become well known, if not infamous for overcrowding and less than sanitary conditions. When the children arrived we, the medical team, quickly triaged the migrants, separating those who may be seriously ill from those with minor complaints. It quickly became apparent that, unlike earlier groups, many of the migrants could not stop itching. As good doctors we began creating a differential diagnosis. Could this be: atopic dermatitis, contact dermatitis, scabies or something unique to the tropical origin of our patients, such as leishmaniasis or cutaneous larvae migrans? Many of the children had extremely itchy red bumps and blisters covering their upper arms and trunks; some of the younger children and infants had lesions on their feet (soles) and palms of their hands. Examination of these lesions led to the diagnosis. All of our patients had fine, linear, slightly scaly lines about 0.5cm to 1cm on the webs of their fingers and many had these lines on their neck, axillae and feet. Curiously, many of their mothers asked us for cebollas (onions). These mothers would cut the onions in half and rub the child's lesions with the freshly cut side of the onion. They informed us that this was 'tratamiento' (treatment) for their 'infección en la piel' (skin infection). Unfortunately, scabies became one more challenge and delay in the very long journey these weary mothers and their exhausted children had undertaken.

Immigration

Of course, scabies amongst immigrant populations is nothing new. Emma Lazarus's sonnet written to raise funds for the Statue of Liberty pedestal describes conditions that would seem to be rather favourable to the scabies mite:

> Give me your tired, your poor,
> Your huddled masses yearning to breathe free,
> The wretched refuse of your teeming shore.
> Send these, the homeless, tempest-tossed to me,
> I lift my lamp beside the golden door.

Utilizing immigrants as scapegoats is also not a new phenomenon. A considerable increase in scabies cases on the large East Coast cities in the late-nineteenth century led authorities to point their fingers at immigrants arriving en masse on American shores.[11] These immigrants hailed from Eastern and Southern Europe in disproportionately higher numbers than their prior counterparts, and thus were targets of derision by the Anglo-Saxon establishment (112). In 1893 the Philadelphia dermatologist H.W. Stelwagon wrote:

Of first importance is the character of recent immigration. It is common knowledge that the present immigrant is, on the average, far below the standard in cleanliness etc., that obtained some years ago, and this extremely undesirable class, largely made up of Russians, Poles, Huns, and Italians, have, especially for the past eight or ten years, been arriving here in great numbers. (111)

Cramped third-class shipping conditions, also known as 'steerage', increased the likelihood of contracting scabies on the trans-Atlantic voyage. While first- and second-class passengers enjoyed private cabins, steerage passengers were crammed together by the hundreds in tight and often filthy conditions, ideal for spreading scabies. 'Many of those even who are free from the disease when embarking, are fairly certain to acquire it on their way over', Stelwagon wrote. He proceeded to advocate that immigrants with scabies be refused entry until they received treatment, writing, 'There is absolutely no reason that an immigrant with the itch be allowed to land.' This, however, required that resources be devoted to identifying those affected with The Itch in the first place.

By 1917, scabies was one of a long list of many diagnosis that immigration officers at Ellis Island were instructed to screen for.[12] Line inspection, where steerage-class immigrants were subject to 'examination' was a hurried and random process, far from ideal for diagnosing scabies. The average inspector was expected to examine between two to five thousand passengers per day, with immigrants receiving an even more cursory inspection on busy days when many ships had arrived (114). Typically only seconds were available to assess if an immigrant had a multitude of diseases, scabies included. It thus goes without saying that scabies cases easily escaped medical detection (194). From here, immigrants would carry The Itch to their new communities, where, often living in cramped quarters, they could additionally spread it. Depending on the various ethnic composition of neighbourhoods, scabies became variably known as 'the Polish itch', 'the Italian itch', 'the Hungarian itch', and so forth (110).

War

Of all the human activities favourable for the spread of scabies, war ranks at the very top of the list. In conditions of wartime, the mite benefits from soldiers living in close quarters, from the mass movement and dislocation of populations, and from poverty and a general lack of medical resources. Friedman wrote:

It is … no exaggeration to say that there never has been an extended war in which the unwelcome acarus did not actively, joyously, and in great numbers participate. Indeed it may truly be said of the itch mite, that ever since wars began its role always has been that of a voraciously belligerent neutral, getting under the skin of and making life miserable for the soldiers of both sides, with fine impartiality. (14)

Scabies and its attendant itch have likely plagued armies in battle since pre-historic times. Convincing documentation of The Itch complicating the the-atre of war dates back to at least eighteenth-century Europe. Thus it should come as no surprise that despite a general confusion amongst physicians and scientists as to the origin of The Itch, military men were comparatively ad-vanced in their knowledge. As fighting effectiveness depended on the health of their troops, the military took the subject seriously. The military physician Sir John Pringle, regarded as one of the fathers of military medicine, wrote very eruditely about scabies in his 1753 Treatise *Observations of the Diseases of the Army in Camp and Garrison*. In this work he devoted an entire chapter to The Itch, demonstrating remarkable knowledge regarding its cause, control, and treatment (77).[13] He specifically distinguished scabies from another military scourge, scurvy, writing:

and, that tho' both the scurvy and itch may coincide on board our ships, yet they are to be considered as two distinct ailments; the first arising from the foul air and bad provisions; and the other, from the uncleanliness of the men and contagion; each requiring a different cure.

Across the Atlantic, scabies was also wreaking havoc on warring armies. Prior to the American Revolutionary War, it had been commonplace in the colonies. Advertisements for scabies treatment could be noted in newspapers of the day, including the *Pennsylvania Gazette*, published by a young Benjamin Franklin, which in 1731 promoted an 'ointment for the ITCH' (Figure 5.2).

Meanwhile, Benjamin Rush, a signee of the Declaration of Independence and physician and Professor of Medicine at the University of Pennsylvania, advo-cated treating the 'inveterate itch' through old school Galenistic techniques of bloodletting and purging. Scabies is known to have been widespread amongst the continental army whilst at their winter camp Valley Forge. General George Washington, at the advice of his doctors, even had separate huts constructed for housing and treating of scabietic soldiers (116).

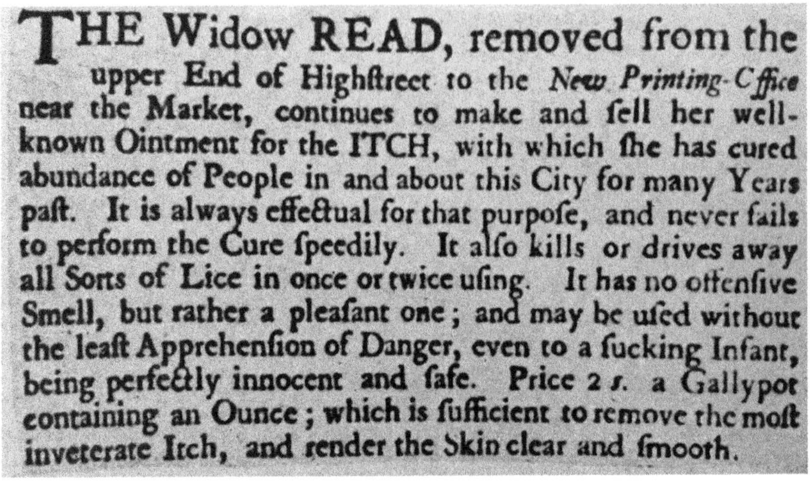

THE Widow READ, removed from the upper End of Highftreet to the *New Printing-Cffice* near the Market, continues to make and fell her well-known Ointment for the ITCH, with which fhe has cured abundance of People in and about this City for many Years paft. It is always effectual for that purpofe, and never fails to perform the Cure fpeedily. It alfo kills or drives away all Sorts of Lice in once or twice ufing. It has no offenfive Smell, but rather a pleafant one; and may be ufed without the leaft Apprehenfion of Danger, even to a fucking Infant, being perfectly innocent and fafe. Price 2 *s.* a Gallypot containing an Ounce; which is fufficient to remove the moft inveterate Itch, and render the Skin clear and fmooth.

Figure 5.2 An advertisement from Benjamin Franklin's *Pennsylvania Gazette* (1731) suggesting that The Itch was a common problem in colonial America.

Interestingly, after the American Revolutionary War, The Itch became rare in the newly independent United States of America, and soon faded from collective memory.[14] Two generations later, American dermatologists, unless they had trained in Europe, were largely unfamiliar with its diagnosis (70). As a result, when scabies resurged in the American Civil War, it was not readily recognized. Called army itch or camp itch, it soon became an overwhelming scourge. It has been estimated that more than 10% of all Union soldiers were affected (54). A variety of theories as to its cause were put forth, amongst them poor hygiene. One of General Lee's surgeons blamed camp itch on the severe shortage of soap. In 1864 he wrote to Confederate president Jefferson Davis to report that 'the soap ration for this Army has become a serious question ... the great want of cleanliness ... is now producing sickness among the men in the trenches.' There was, however, the occasional medic who recognized the condition as scabies and was able to cure it with appropriate treatment. One such individual was Surgeon Lunsford Pitts Yandell Jr of the 4th Tennessee Regimen. He observed many cases of 'army itch' amongst his fellow Confederate soldiers. He wrote that army itch was in fact scabies, often with secondary impetigo or other infectious complications, and recounted how he himself succumbed:

In 1862, in the Confederate service, I became the subject of *Sarcoptes hominis*. At the same time several generals and some very elegant ladies of my acquaintance were my fellow sufferers. At first the itching was not only not unpleasant, but was positively delightful .... Very soon, however, the pruritus became terrific. I often awoke at night exhausted and panting from violent scratching begun in my sleep. I lacerated the skin with my nails to abate the tortured itching, for the smarting pain of the abraded surface was far preferable to the pruritus. Sulfur ointment relieved me entirely in three days.

For the Confederate army, the problem with sulphur, a treatment for scabies since antiquity, was in procuring it. Because sulphur constituted an integral component of gunpowder, the Northern naval blockade led to it being in very short supply. Confederate doctors thus were thus relegated to searching for alternative therapies to treat 'camp itch' (187). Experimentation with local flora and fauna led to the use of many natural products as treatment. Among these were the poke root (*Phytolacca decandra*), broom straw (*Andropagon virginicus*), and slipper elm (*Ulmus rubra*), as well as an ointment made from the inner bark of the elderberry tree (*Sambucus sp.*). Likely these concoctions were of variable efficacy. A similar strategy of exploiting the products of nature for their antimite properties in the twentieth century would eventually yield the discovery of permethrin, which today, as a cream, is considered a first-line treatment for scabies in many countries (54).

As soldiers returned home from the Civil War battlefields, army itch or camp itch, spread to others, reaching epidemic proportions. While the origin of this strange skin disease baffled many, the dermatologist James White, who had trained in Vienna with von Hebra, was not fooled:

I have examined a great many cases of 'army itch' in returned soldiers and their families, and do not hesitate to express the opinion that it is simply scabies ... the soldiers brought it home with them on furlough and after discharge from service, and thus it became a widespread epidemic affecting all classes of society.[15]

Only when scabies reared its head in World War I did military personnel embark on a more systematic approach to understanding it. The nature of trench warfare with close crowding and attendant filth resulted in a large number of diseases attributable to animal parasites, especially body lice and scabies. The resulting infections that occurred in soldiers who had scratched their skin into open and festering wounds could be debilitating and even life-threatening, especially in the preantibiotic era. Often the pyodermic, or infectious, complications of scabies would manifest as impetigo, or boils, most prominent on the buttocks, elbows, and knees. Sometime these could be so severe as to

thoroughly mask the scabietic nature of the eruption itself. The military physicians H. MacCormac and W.D. Small described the British experience in
World War I, writing in 1917:

> Of the skin diseases found amongst soldiers—excluding pediculosis [lice],
> scabies is by far the commonest. When uncomplicated, its effects incapaci-
> tate a man but little; but in consequence of the hard conditions of active ser-
> vice, secondary pyodermic complications are frequent and severe, and these
> are a very real cause of prolonged sickness. In contrast to three or four days
> required for the complete cure of a simple case we have found that when
> pyodermic complications are established the period necessary is greatly
> prolonged—the average stay in hospital over larger number of cases being
> 31.67 days. (23)

In World War I, approximately 40% of skin diseases requiring treatment in the
American expeditionary force were due to scabies (14). Prior to the advent of
penicillin, which could cure skin infections caused by heavy scratching, scabies and its infective complications ravaged the armies fighting in Northern
Europe.[16] In place of antibiotics, military physicians were forced to treat their
sickened comrades with rudimentary and ineffective preparations. Impetigo
and pustular outbreaks were most effectively treated with ammoniated mercury ointment, while boils were treated with ichthyol ointment, both of which
have been largely discarded from modern medicine (6).

The problem was severe enough that the British War office tasked Captain
J.W. Munro of the Royal Army Medical Corps 'to obtain a knowledge of the life
history and habits of the mite causing scabies in the army, to ascertain its mode
of spread and to improve the existing methods or, where necessary, to devise
new methods of dealing with it, based on that knowledge' (14). Munro had
studied zoology as an undergraduate, and subsequently earned a doctorate in
forestry. He was performing further scientific investigation at Imperial College
in London when he was redirected to the 1st Eastern General Hospital and
Quick Laboratory at Cambridge to study military aspects of lice and scabies.
Mincing no words, Munro's initial observation was that 'no two accounts of
the life history of the mite agree and there is a similar difference of opinion
regarding its mode of spread or dispersal'. In one contemporary account of
the time, scabies was attributable to factors as variable as blankets and under-
clothing, mangy horses, and infected women (23).

Munro, in the course of his studies, made many pioneering observations,
and laid the foundation for the future ground-breaking work of Mellanby in

the following World War. Munro was among the first to attempt to propagate mites in the laboratory away from the human body. This did not prove to be an easy task, as skin samples removed from the body and handled in the laboratory dried quickly and provided a poor substrate for scabies. Yet the same skin samples, when kept artificially hydrated, swelled up, becoming spongy and equally unsuitable. Munro admitted that all his attempts to set up a laboratory, or in vitro, system to study the mite away from the human body had ended in failure. Others have subsequently tried and failed as well, a shortcoming that limits our ability to make progress in scabies research to this day.[17]

Munro found that he could extract female mites out of their burrows using a dissecting needle and confine them at various alternate skin sites using a glass ring held directly on the skin with elastic bands. When he transferred a female mite in this fashion to an area not typically inhabited, such as the forearm, Munro noted it would burrow into the skin superficially for protection. However when the glass ring was removed, within several hours, the mite would vacate its temporary shelter and migrate to preferred sites, which Munro concluded were the finger web spaces, inner aspect of the wrists, elbows, uppermost folds of armpits, penis, scrotum, buttocks, back of the knee, ankles, and toes.

Munro tried to isolate and work with the larval and nymphal immature forms of scabies, but found them to be highly delicate and quick to shrivel up and dry out. He was one of the first to make the observation that the scabies mite survived longer under humid conditions. He additionally recognized that mites were more active under conditions of warmth. Prior authors had noted that scabies tended to be itchier at night-time, attributing this to the mite having a nocturnal lifecycle. Munro countered that this nocturnal irritation was rather due to the increased activity of the mite given the warmth it experiences in bundled-up night-time conditions. He wrote:

> The irritation in scabies is most felt by the patient when he is warm and this is due to the fact that the acarus is then most active. That the mite is nocturnal in its habits, a statement common to many authors, is not in accordance with my experience which is that the mite is most active when its host is warm and resting, irrespective of the time of day or night. (22)[18]

He additionally attributed the itchiness experienced in scabies to acrid fluid secreted by the acarus. He dismissed any idea that itchiness was due to sensing the mite wandering around on the skin, as patients sometimes claim, writing, 'I have repeatedly allowed larvae and adult acari to crawl on various parts of my body and have never felt the slightest irritation.'

Munro's extensive scabies investigation also included a series of infectivity experiments that foreshadowed Mellanby's more extensive work to come.[19] Munro had healthy volunteers sleep in a bed that a heavily infested patient had slept in the prior night and described that in a minority of the experiments scabies could be contracted from infested bedding. He additionally performed contagion experiments with clothing and undergarments and wound up coming to the opposite conclusion that Mellanby arrived at 20 years later, finding that inanimate articles (fomites) had the potential to transmit scabies.

Munro summarized his scabies investigation in an erudite 41-page report published in 1919 in the *Journal of the Royal Army Medical Corps*.[20] He concluded that in a military setting, the diagnosis of scabies was best made by noting the following: (i) burrows, (ii) mites on the wrists or penis, and/or (iii) crusted lesions on the buttocks. However, as many soldiers with scabies presented in a highly scratched-up and infected fashion, the detection of burrows, the tell-tale sign of scabies, was often not possible. This presentation of heavily scratched up and infected scabietic soldiers was not dissimilar to that of the many soldiers suffering from body lice. The key difference was the scabies unlike lice had a predilection for the penis, and thus genital inspection was paramount in properly diagnosing scabies. His contemporary MacCormac summed up this sentiment, writing that 'any system of regimental inspection, for the detection of scabies, must permit of an examination of the whole body and above all the penis'. Even today, penile examination can sometimes yield the best (or only) clues that the sufferer of an itchy rash is afflicted with scabies.

Meanwhile away from the lab, scabies thrived in the cramped trench warfare conditions of World War I. Special scabies centres and hospitals were established to control the outbreak amongst troops. After the war was concluded, numerous cases of scabies amongst military men filtered back into the civilian population. During demobilization of American troops in 1919, James Mitchell described the lack of attention to scabies amongst the illnesses of the armed forces, writing:

> In the army, there seems to have been a lamentable failure on the part of medical officers to recognize scabies, judging from the large numbers of infected men who passed through the demobilization camps ... At Camp Pike ... no apparent attempt to treat these men was made. The weights and measures of the men were carefully made and tabulated, but cases of ringworm and scabies by the thousand passed through the station and were returned to civil life to infect the civil population. As a result of the carelessness of the medical examining board of the Army, ringworm of the crotch and scabies will be

disseminated throughout the nation, and will cause great discomfort in the civil population for years to come. (14)

An identical transfer of scabies to the civilian population also occurred in Europe. In 1922, French dermatologist and venereologist Georges Thibierge wrote, 'the increase in the number of cases of scabies, hardly noticeable in the feminine population in the first year of the war, became sharply augmented in the autumn of 1915 when a great number of soldiers, contaminated by promiscuity at the front, returned to Paris'. As Friedman put it, 'the civil population was now suffering dermatologically from the war' (14). At the Hôpital St. Louis in Paris, the number of annual cases of scabies more than doubled. In Vienna a specialized clinic to address this problem was created and called 'The Institute for the Rapid Cure of Scabies'.

Eventually the number of scabies cases decreased in the interwar period, but a noticeable uptick in cases in Britain was noted starting in 1936 and continuing until 1941. Some attributed this to the crowded conditions of 'shelter life'.[21] By the end of 1941, it was estimated that between one to two million individuals were infected with scabies in Britain alone. A similar increase was documented in France (14). Again, the military impact of scabies was felt.[22] In 1942, 72,000 cases of scabies were recorded in British armed forces, with those affected out of active service for an average 4 days (10). It was estimated that this amounted to the equivalent of 800 men being out of commission for one whole year (60).

Notes

1. In a mid-1950s survey of American dermatologists, it was noted that scabies had become 'so rare that it is difficult to maintain index of suspicion', that it was 'difficult to find a case in clinic to demonstrate to students', and 'if you diagnose a rash as scabies, you're probably wrong' (49). To be able to diagnose scabies with confidence, it has been estimated that a practitioner needs to have seen 5–10 cases of scabies during their training (184).
2. The one country where it is, and consistently has been, reportable is Denmark.
3. Of note, the contemporaneous meaning of this term, having been borrowed from medical entomology, now refers to the ennui that comes, to some, after being married for 7 years. The 1955 film with the same name, starring Marilyn Monroe, was based on the 1952 stage play by George Axelrod, who apparently named it so after hearing a comedian recite, 'I know she's over 21 because she's had the seven-year itch four times!'
4. 'Whole regimens of soldiers, the moment they were encamped for the night, threw off their knapsacks and scratched en masse' (117).

5. Dr Friedman devoted a whole book, entitled *The Emperor's Itch*, to the question of whether Napoleon himself had scabies (21). Apocryphally he contracted it when as an artillery commander he assumed control of the cannon whose gunner was suffering from scabies and had just been shot. The act of reloading the cannon with the ramrod multiple times was supposedly the method by which Napoleon contracted The Itch, from which he suffered for many years after. Dr Friedman relates the following quatrain (supposedly from the pen of Ecouchard-Lebrun (117)):

> *Un jour Napoléon me prenant par la main / Cette faveur est sans égale/Dit 'de moi vous aurez quelque chose demain' / Le lendemain j'avais la gale.*

6. Several early print examples include 'Seven Years ITCH Cured!', printed in the *Portland (ME) Gazette* on 25 October 1815 and 'taken with perfect safety, by all ages, for the cure of the following diseases.... also, that corruption so commonly known to the western country as the scab or seven year itch'. from Dr John Mason's Indian Vegetable Panacea, advertised in the *Ohio Statesman* of 26 March 1839.

7. Interestingly, this is particularly seen in Australian Aborigines.

8. Analysis of Israeli Defense Forces records over the course of nearly 20 years, where scabies is a mandatorily reported condition, revealed that nearly 30% more scabies cases were reported in the winter than the summer (3). Similar seasonal periodicity is not seen in tropical climates, where extreme cold is uncommon (174).

9. Scanning electron microscopic studies reveal trails of bacteria in scabies burrows (102).

10. As reported in the *El Paso Times* and *New York Times*:

> Since the Border Patrol opened its station in Clint, Tex., in 2013, it was a fixture in this West Texas farm town.... Most people around Clint had little idea of what went on inside. Agents came and went in pickup trucks; buses pulled into the gates with the occasional load of children apprehended at the border, four miles south. But inside the secretive site that is now on the front lines of the southwest border crisis, the men and women who work there were grappling with the stuff of nightmares. Outbreaks of scabies, shingles and chickenpox were spreading among the hundreds of children and adults who were being held in cramped cells, agents said. (172)

11. Friedman pointed out, at the time of the first meeting of the American Dermatological Association in 1876 in Philadelphia, scabies was not discussed, and there were no records of even a single case (14). Part of this may be in fact have been due to ignorance, as familiarity with scabies amongst American dermatologists was largely limited to the select few who had been trained abroad.

12. In some instances, US medical offers examined passengers in various ports of Europe prior to disembarkation. Stephen Graham booked passage on the Cunard liner from Liverpool to New York in 1913, and described his experience:

> There were fifteen hundred of us; each man and woman, still carrying handbags and baskets, filed past a doctor and two assistants, and was cursorily examined for diseases of the eye or skin. 'Hats and gloves off!' was our first greeting on the liner. We marched slowly up to the medical trio, and each one as he passed had his eyelid seized by the doctor and turned inside out with a little instrument. It was a strange liberty to take with one's person; but doctors are getting their own way nowadays, and they were looking for trachoma. For the rest the passing of hands through our hair and examination of our skin for signs of scabies was not so rough, and the cleaner-looking people were not molested. (137)

13. Pringle in his first edition, wrote:

[The Itch] is also of a contagious nature, but the infection is only communicated by the contact of a foul person, his cloaths, bedding, etc, and not by effluvia, as in the dysentery and malignant fever. It is confined to the skin and seems best accounted for by Leeuwenhoek, from certain small insects he discovered in pustules by the microscope.

In his second edition, he added:

Since the first edition was published, I have seen a paper in the Phil. Transact. for the year 1703 called, 'An abstract of a letter from Dr. Bonomo to Signior Redi' containing some observations concerning the worms of human bodies by Dr. Richard Mead. By which account I find that Dr. Bonomo was the first that discovered these animalcula and likewise proposed of curing the itch by externals only.

14. Likely though, it did not fully disappear. In the 1850s, a condition known as prairie itch (also termed prairie dig, Illinois itch, Western itch, or Missouri mange) had been reported in Midwestern states and territories, and likely represents pre–Civil War scabies.

15. White further expounded:

During the period of my [student] years passed in the Tremont Medical School, and the lecture seasons of the University, 1853-1856, I do not remember to have seen a case; so that I might have entered practice after receiving the degree of doctor of medicine without being able to recognize the disease. In the immediate continuation of my study in Europe, where the disease was almost a normal condition of life among the lower classes, and where, in the vast standing armies, soldiers were treated for the affection by the regiment at a time, abundant opportunity offered to become familiar with it in all its possible manifestations. On my return I found that it did occur more frequently than it was recognized amongst us, although rarely. But with the breaking out of the war of the Rebellion, three years subsequently, it became after a time very prevalent among the soldiers, probably through the enlistment of recent immigrants and the favoring conditions of camp life, and later was established as a general epidemic in our armies over their vast field of operations. But so little were army and volunteer surgeons acquainted with the disease and its management that they regarded it as an unknown affection 'defying nomenclature and classification'. (107)

16. Captain Frank Knowles summed up the gravity in 1918, writing, 'There is probably no greater problem today in the fighting forces in Europe than the group of animal parasitic diseases'. (6)

17. As previously mentioned, in recent years a porcine (pig) model of scabies has been established. (42)

18. Munro additionally described the role of warmth in burrowing:

During January and February the writer carried out a number of experiments to test the rate of burrowing of the females. The acari were placed on the wrist and allowed to burrow in. The laboratory temperature was low and, in all instances but one, the females concealed themselves under the epidermis until the writer entered a warm room when they commenced burrowing again. If, however, the hand was held over a radiator or other source of heat the mites commenced to burrow and it was possible by alternately warming and cooling the hand affected to regulate the rate of burrowing. Mellanby would later determine that the scabies mite does not move at all once the temperature drops below 16 °C and is at that point in a 'chill coma'. (15, 195)

19. Munro wrote:

The subjects of the experiments were civilians who volunteered for the purpose and received board and lodging and a weekly sum in remuneration. Owing to the limited number of volunteers available and the necessity of curing them for succeeding experiments, and allowing a minimum period of fourteen days to elapse after cure to insure its certainty, the experiments are limited in number and scope, and it is hoped that further experiments on a large scale may be made on these lines. (22)

20. After the war, Munro returned to the subject of forest entomology eventually becoming a professor of entomology at Imperial College in London in 1930, where he studied varied subjects including pest infestation of stored foods on London docks. Future titles written by him would include *Report on Insect Infestation of Stored Cacao*, *Report on a Survey of the Infestation of Grain by Insects*, and *Pests of Stored Products*. His research led to advances in the fumigation industry. He died in 1968 (119).

21. Mellanby did not necessarily agree with this explanation, pointing out that a concomitant increase in scabies was noted in British towns that were not bombed in the Second World War (19).

22. Interestingly no increase in scabies amongst troops was noted in the wars in Vietnam or Korea (31 and refs therein).

6

History

You've Come a Long Way Scaby

Humans have been afflicted by scabies for millennia, though exactly when scabies was recognized as being a disease in its own right is unknown. Creative licence is required to further pinpoint the exact initial documented reference. Various authors have suggested that the Hebrew term 'zaraath', found in the Old Testament (Leviticus 13:8), is a reference to scabies. 'Zaraath' has also been translated into Greek as 'Lepra', which is the origin of the word leprosy. 'Zaraath' is used too loosely from this time period to mean anything more than a scaly skin abnormality, which may have included cases of scabies, leprosy, or other conditions.

The ancient Greeks may have been aware of the scabies mite. Synthesizing the ideas of his time, the philosopher Aristotle (384–322 BC) proposed the concept of spontaneous generation, in which living organisms were believed to derive directly from nonliving matter. This theory helped the ancients explain many natural observed phenomenon. For example, it could explain the explosive outburst of frogs and salamanders on the banks of the Nile, during the annual floods which transformed the parched baked-bricked riverbanks into a muddy mass teeming with life. In his treatise, *Historia Animalium*, Aristotle wrote that lice, bugs, and fleas, generated spontaneously from the decay of human flesh.

In relating details of the louse ($\varphi\theta\epsilon\iota\rho\epsilon\varsigma$), Aristotle described a parasite that we would recognize today. He stated that it was more likely to be found on the heads of children than adults, and that it could even infest many other hair bearing animals as well as birds. Where his description becomes less recognizable, however, is when Aristotle described features sounding much more in keeping with scabies—that the louse '[gave] rise to small clear vesicles which can be opened and removed by a needle'.[1] It is difficult to determine with certainty, but based on this passage, most likely Aristotle and the ancient Greeks were aware of the scabies mite but confused it with the louse, thinking they were one and the same. Confusing these two parasites with each other would be a common mistake up until the sixteenth century, when English physician Thomas Moffet explicitly clarified that they are in fact different pests.

By Roman times, an itchy and scabby skin condition called scabies was widely known. The term '*scabere*' in fact means 'to scrape' or 'to scratch' in Latin. Writings from this time period, however, lack key features that allow us to recognize this condition as clearly being scabies, such as a description of the burrow or a listing of the regions of skin commonly affected. In 25 AD, the Roman author Aulus Cornelius Celsus described scabies in the following fashion that would leave modern day readers scratching their head:

> The scabies is a hardness of the skin, of a muddy color, from whence pustules arise, some of them moist, other dry ... and in these there follows a continued itching ulceration, which in certain cases spreads very fast. In some people it goes entirely off, in others it returns at a certain season of the year.

Amazingly, despite having an incomplete understanding of The Itch, the ancients were able to discover an effective cure for scabies based solely on their observations and empirical treatments. Celsus recommended sulphur mixed with liquid pitch as a remedy for scabies, which undoubtedly was effective. In one form or another, sulphur remained the treatment of choice for scabies for nearly 2000 years. Only in the last several decades has its use lost favour, although it still works when employed. It remains the treatment of choice during pregnancy and breastfeeding.

Did non-Western civilizations know about scabies? Not unexpectedly, the role of non-Western developments in the history of scabies is, and continues to remain, a neglected area of study. The late American dermatologist and pre-eminent twentieth-century historian of scabies Reuben Friedman in 1937 called attention to a passage from the Chinese author Ch'ao Yuan-fang who wrote or helped compile an early medical text entitled *Zhubing Yuanhou Lun* (*General Treatise on the Etiology and Symptoms of Diseases*) dating to the Sui Dynasty (581–618 AD). In it he wrote:

> The itchy scabies sores (jie chuang) always contain a tiny worm. We can extract it with a needle and see its worm-like shape when it is dropped into water ... More often than not jie chuang first appears between the fingers and toes. Babies often acquire it from the mother if she herself is infected. (82, 167)

This passage, like others from antiquity, contains intriguing but also question-able references to scabies. Nevertheless, it should serve as a reminder that the ultimate chapter(s) in the history of scabies remain to be written.

Regardless of precisely when The Itch, as a disease, was first known, and more specifically when the scabies mite was first detected by humans, we can say that by late antiquity, the medical establishment would have assimilated it into its Galenistic world view. Here, scabies like all other illnesses, was attrib-uted to an imbalance of the four body humours: phlegm, blood, yellow bile, and black bile. These represented projections of what the ancient Greeks con-sidered to be the core elements from which all things originated—water, earth, fire, and air (200, 201). At the time, the concept of a parasite causing illness would have been completely foreign.

And in short, for centuries contemporary understanding of scabies revolved around the imbalance of body humours. When eventually confronted with visual proof that a mite could be found in lesions of scabies, physicians and scientists of the day resorted to the Aristotelian concept of spontaneous gen-eration. In the case of scabies, the presence of a mite could thus be explained away as a by-product of diseased tissues. It would take may additional cen-turies for the medical profession to actually accept that the mite itself was in fact what caused scabies.

It is no surprise then that peasants, laypersons, and other commoners, after being subjected to bloodletting, purges, or other debilitating measures, took it upon themselves to find pragmatic yet effective treatments for the disease. In many different regions, peasant women, without fanfare, independently dis-covered that The Itch could be relieved by extracting small specs out of the skin with a needle (125, 182).[2] Such knowledge, where it existed, would be passed down orally, but was dismissed by men of medicine as vulgar.[3]

The earliest unequivocal description of the scabies mite comes from the late Middle Ages, though there is no established consensus as to who was first. Several contenders exist, whose writings have been analysed and debated by early scabologists. The tenth-century Persian physician al-Tabari is one pos-sibility. He wrote a multivolume medical work called *Hippocratic Treatises*. In book seven, he described multiple different variants of scabies. One of them, described as 'bloody scabies', suggests an awareness of the presence of a mite in human skin:

This animalcule can be removed with the point of a needle. If placed on the nail and exposed to the heat of the sun or fire, it moves. If the animalcule is crushed between two fingernails, one hears it crack. This type of scabies is most easily treated. The disease may be cured by administration of laxatives and the killing of the animals.

The other nine variants of scabies that al-Tabari laid forth, however, have little or nothing to do with scabies as we know it, thus betraying the idea that he had any real understanding of the topic (206).[4]

Another possible candidate for earliest positive identification of the scabies mite comes from the Moorish physician Abu Merwan Abdelmalik ben Sohr (Avenzoar) of Cordova (b. 1070 Spain, d. 1162 Morocco) whose posthumous work, *Directions to Successful Medical Cure and Dietetic Treatment* (1165), contains the following description: 'There is something called soab which bores into the body from without; it lives under the skin, and if the skin is scratched in certain spots a tiny animal comes out, which is hardly visible to the naked eye.'

Other Arabic texts of the same time, however, describe soab as animals living between the hairs, which are transferable by combing—a description immediately recognizable as the head louse. Similar to Aristotle, it seems possible that Avenzoar may have in part confused scabies with lice. Yet the specifics of his description—that soab lives under the skin, bores into the body, and is hardly visible to the naked eye—seem much more in keeping with the description of the acarus rather than a louse.

von Hebra considered Saint Hildegarde (1098–1179) the first to indisputably describe the scabies mite. Saint Hildegarde, the abbess of Rupertsberg Convent, located in modern day Germany, wrote a compendium of herbal remedies entitled *Physika*, where the following passage can be found:

> There is another mint which is large; it is hot rather than cold. This should be crushed and placed above and around the place where the Suren or Snevelzen are hurting the person with their nibbling; and they will die, as the coldness of this same mentha major is rather bitter, and therefore kills the above-mentioned little worms, which are born in the human flesh.

Despite our inability to pinpoint exactly when scabies was first described, by the end of the Middle Ages, clear references to the presence of a mite in the lesions of The Itch had appeared. The medieval thirteenth-century French poem on chivalry, *Romance of the Roses*, mentions that women should tend to the appearance of their hands and, if needed, remove any 'sirons' with a needle (or else wear gloves).[5] There is evidence to suggest that Shakespeare was aware of scabies when in *Romeo and Juliet* he wrote about 'worms pricked from the fingers of a lazy maid' (126). As far as physicians were concerned, some seemed to know about the presence of a mite in the skin as well. The fourteenth-century French physician Guy de Chauliac described small animals that were conta-gious in nature, 'which make winding paths by gnawing between the skin and flesh [*carnem & cutum*], especially in the hands of persons of leisure' (125). In a work published in 1533, Alexander Benedictus, who had been professor at Padua, at the time a part of the Republic of Venice, described the scabies mite as being smaller than a lentil seed, which creeps under the skin, especially in children, but rarely on their heads. In 1557 the Italian physician Scaliger and in 1577 French physician Joubertus wrote of a method for extracting mites with a needle. The renowned physician and surgeon Ambrose Pare in sixteenth-century Paris wrote, 'the mites are little animals, always hidden under the skin, there they crawl and gnaw the skin, little by little, exciting a disagreeable itching. They can be extracted with pins or needles.' Thus it is quite clear that by the beginning of the Renaissance, the cause of scabies was understood and known in certain learned circles.

The sixteenth-century English physician Thomas Moffet (1553–1604) was the first to clearly describe the scabies mite as being distinct from the louse (149). Moffet named the scabies mite 'acari', borrowing the Aristotelian term 'akari'—meaning the smallest 'indivisible' animal. Moffet's 'acari' was meant to refer to one mite; however, the term was later assumed to be plural. And from the assumed plural 'acari', the singular form of the noun 'acarus' was derived (8). He likely observed the scabies mite using a handheld magnifying lens, though he did not leave behind a drawing or diagram (148, 149). Moffet de-scribed such mites as being found on humans, as well as in cheese, and wax, and termed the scabies mite as a 'wheale worm', which moves along 'without hardly any feet'. Moffet correctly noted that the scabies mite doesn't live in the actual pustule seen in scabies themselves but rather 'hard bye' (nearby). While somewhat cryptic, this is the first recorded suggestion that the scabies mite was not to be found in the pustules or blister bumps located at the origination or entrance of the scabietic burrow. His findings were summarized and written by the year 1590, but his final work, *Insectorum sive Minimorum Animalium Theatrum*, was only belatedly and posthumously published in 1634. It was sub-sequently translated into English with under title *The Theater of Insects or of Lesser Living Creatures.*

Moffet's description of where the mite doesn't reside carries great import-ance. Starting around this time period, physicians seeking to determine the cause of The Itch would investigate the contents of the pustules of scabies.[6] This would be a logical choice, as the pustules would be one of the more prominent features of The Itch, certainly more so than any subtle adjacent burrow. And in this pustule, inevitably they would be unable to find a mite.[7] Given today's knowledge, this makes good sense, as we know the mite resides not in the pustule, an immunological reaction and sideshow, but rather at the leading edge of the burrow. However at the time, this was not widely recognized. Those specifically questioning the idea that a mite could be the cause of The Itch would search the pustule and come up empty. They would thus arrive at the erroneous conclusion that mites in fact were not the cause of The Itch. Understandably, this led to confusion and impaired the general understanding of scabies for several additional centuries.

In spite of such missteps, science would eventually unravel the mysteries of The Itch. The minute size of the mite was certainly a limiting factor when the most advanced technology for visualization was the magnifying glass. Thus the development of the microscope in the early seventeenth century allowed for considerable advances in the understanding of scabies to be made. Using an early and rudimentary microscope in 1657, the Dresden physician August Hauptmann (1607–1674) published the first-known sketch of the scabies mite, or any microscopic organism for that matter (148). This appeared in his treatise, *The Ancient Wolkenstein Hot Bathe and Water Cures*, in which Hauptmann wrote on the curative nature of the ancient natural springs in the area. A variety of patients came to these springs seeking cures for their ailments. Presumably patients with scabies benefitted from the sulphur or sulphite content. Hauptmann's drawing shows an oval appearing insect having three pairs of legs and two pairs of long terminal bristles (Figure 6.1).

While technically inadequate in some details, its immediately likeness to a female mite enables us to deduce without hesitation that humans have been able to positively identify scabies under the microscope for more than 350 years. At the time, however, very few were aware of his drawing, and even those who were would have regarded it as a curiosity at best. But by the middle of the seventeenth century, select scientists and naturalists had with their own eyes observed the presence of a tiny mite in the itchy skin eruption that we would term 'scabies', even if they were a small minority.

Amongst the medical profession, the term 'scabies' gained wide circulation but was used rather loosely to describe a variety of itchy afflictions. It assumed various regional names: '*Seuren*' in Germany, '*Sierken*' in the Netherlands, '*Sarna*' and '*Asturias*' in Iberia, '*Cyrons*' in France, '*Siro*' and '*Sciri*' in Piedmont, '*Brigant*' in Gascony, '*Rogne*' in Provence, '*Pellicello*' in Tuscany and the Venetian republic, and '*Handwyrm*' in England. Many of these words appear to originate from '*chirones*', the Greek word for hand (Χείρων). Despite advances in microscopy, the prevailing intellectual framework of scabies

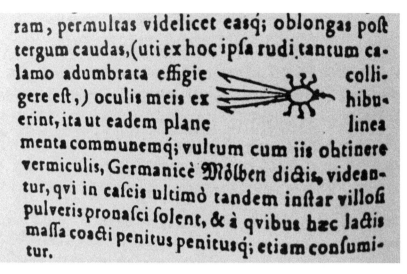

ram, permultas videlicet easq; oblongas poſt tergum caudas,(uti ex hoc ipſa rudi tantum ca-lamo adumbrata effigie colli-gere eſt,) oculis meis ex hibu-erint, ita ut eadem plane linea menta communemq; vultum cum iis obtinere vermiculis, Germanicè Mölben dictis, videan-tur, qvi in caſcis ultimò tandem inſtar villoſi pulveris pronaſci ſolent, & à qvibus hæc lactis maſſa coacti penitus penitusq; etiam conſumi-tur.

Figure 6.1 The first-known depiction of the scabies mite, or any infectious organism for that matter. Drawn in 1657 by the Dresden physician August Hauptmann (1607–1674), it depicts a creature with three pairs of legs and two pairs of terminal bristles. Likely Hauptmann observed a female mite, and the first set of anal bristles are in fact the fourth pair of legs which terminate in bristles.
Reproduced from Friedman, Reuben. (1947). *The Story of Scabies*, Vol 1. New York: Froben Press.

remained for the most part unchanged as it had been over the prior centuries. Scabies, like other diseases, continued to be attributed to foul humours circulating in the body. Girolamo Mercuriale, professor of medicine at University of Padua, in one of the first medical works ever dedicated to skin disease, *De Morbis Cutaneis*, gives us good insight into how scabies was conceptualized. Mercuriale divided scabies into two forms, dry and moist scabies, writing in 1572: 'The basis of scabies is in the blood; this may be concluded from the fact that scabies involves the entire body, and no body fluid is so diffusely distributed as the blood; the blood of scabies is not pure but thick … purulent, or biliously salted.'

Mercuriale concluded that the vile humours of scabies could transmit from the blood to the skin, and to this he attributed the contagiousness and communicability of scabies. Physicians of the day thus actually discouraged the treatment of scabies with topical medications, fearing that it would drive the disease back into the body where it could cause more serious harm to internal organs. Bloodletting or internal ingestion of medication was thus viewed as the appropriate treatment. As summarized by the English physician Thomas Spooner in the early 1700s, 'He that would cure The Itch … must first of all cleanse the blood.'

Within Renaissance Europe, knowledge of scabies was most advanced in the Italian city states. An early compendium of the Italian language, the *Vocabulario dell'Academia della Crusca* (1612), lists 'pellicello' as a tiny worm which arises in the skin of patients and produces an intense itching. This was the intellectual milieu in which the Italians Giovanni Cosimo Bonomo (1663–1696) and Diacinto Cestoni (1637–1718) produced the first comprehensive and convincing description of the scabies mite and the disease it causes, in the form of a letter addressed to the Italian naturalist Francesco Redi (1626–1697) (Figure 6.2).

Bonomo and Cestoni's letter of 1687[8] is a landmark document which deserves to be reprinted in detail, but first a few words about Bonomo and Cestoni are warranted.

Bonomo was a physician who undertook medical training in Pisa, and spent time working as a ship physician on slave galleys in Livorno, a bustling city on the Tuscan coast. In this setting he had the opportunity to closely observe a variety of infectious disease amongst men living in close quarters. One of these

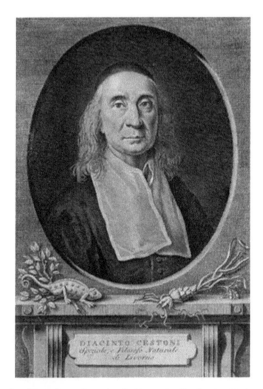

Figure 6.2 Sketch of Diacinto Cestoni (1637–1718) who in conjunction with Giovanni Cosimo Bonomo (1663–1696) 'discovered' the acarian origin of scabies. No extant sketch of Bonomo is known to exist.

appears to have been scabies. He observed men, either on ships or in public bathhouses, or perhaps both, removing minute specks of material out of others skin to relieve their itch (Figure 6.3).

He also had occasion to witness poor peasant women extracting mites with a needle from the skin of children who were affected by scabies. He would not be the first nor the last pioneer of scabies to have originally witnessed such extractions by villagers or laypersons. Bonomo decided to investigate what exactly was being removed from these patients. To assist him he recruited Cestoni, an apothecary, noted naturalist, and colleague of his father. Aside from being a pharmacy, Cestoni's locale was a forum for learned men to meet. Unusual for the day, Cestoni possessed a microscope[9] and good technical skill in using it. It was the combination of Bonomo's astute clinical observations and Cestoni's technical skill allowed them to come up with their ground-breaking findings.

Their repeated examination of material removed from patients with The Itch led them to confidently conclude that the disease scabies was caused by a mite. Moreover, on at least one occasion, they observed a mite laying an egg. They deduced that the scabies mite lived and behaved like an insect. Different sexes mated and the female laid eggs, thereby propagating the lifecycle. Perhaps not immediately obvious, but very noteworthy, was that this theory required no

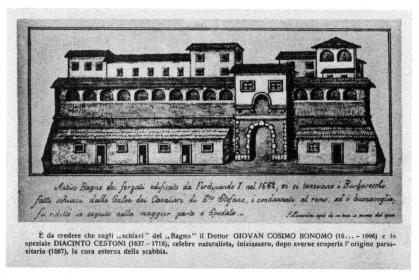

È da credere che sugli „schiavi" del „Bagno" il Dottor GIOVAN COSIMO BONOMO (16... – 1696) e lo speziale DIACINTO CESTONI (1637 – 1718), celebre naturalista, iniziassero, dopo averne scoperta l' origine parassitaria (1687), la cura esterna della scabbia.

Figure 6.3 The Bagno or public bathhouse in Leghorne, known today as Livorno. Leghorn was a bustling port of commerce during Renaissance Italy and it was in such a bathhouse that Bonomo described first observing persons extracting the, scabies mite out of the skin.

need to invoke Aristotle's concept of spontaneous generation. Mites lived in the skin where they procreated and thus accordingly caused the skin disease known as scabies, and not because they had generated from decomposing tissue.

To help disseminate their findings, Bonomo and Cestoni sought out the renowned Tuscan naturalist Francesco Redi (1626–1697), as specifically someone who would lend a sympathetic ear (Figure 6.4).

Redi held favour in the court of the Grand Duke of Tuscany and was a prominent scientist. Today he is widely considered to be the father of experimental biology. His statue currently stands in the Uffizi Gallery in Florence. Amongst his accomplishments, he was the first person to question the theory of spontaneous generation through actual experimentation. Redi derived inspiration for his experiments from observing that butchers and commoners routinely protected meat in the summer by covering it with white cloth. Redi thus created a simple experimental setup where flies either had direct access to rotting meat at the bottom of glass jars or did not because of the presence of a thin layer of

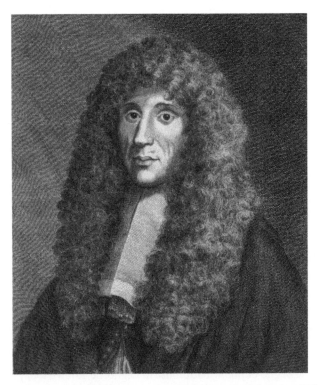

Figure 6.4 A sketch of the Italian naturalist Francesco Redi (1626-1697), a widely respected scientist of his day who helped debunk the theory of spontaneous generation which had held currency since antiquity.

gauze placed on the top of the jar. Maggots only subsequently developed on the meat which flies had direct access to. From this, Redi made the radical proposal that 'All life comes from life' (*Omne vivum ex vivo*).

Bonomo and Cestoni penned a letter to Redi describing their scabies observations on 20 June 1687. Redi apparently viewed Bonomo and Cestoni's findings with scepticism but nevertheless appreciated the careful and original nature of their observations, and holding both of these individuals in high regard, he decided to disseminate their findings in a small pamphlet. To make this pamphlet more publication worthy, Redi embellished Bonomo and Cestoni's descriptions, as well as added his own observations on cockroaches, woodworms, beetles, caterpillars, and other insects, more than doubling its length. Ironically, Redi's additions are of no interest today, and are universally omitted when discussing this important document. On 18 July 1687, *Osservazioni intorno a' pellicelli del corpo umano* was published in Florence in the form of a pamphlet containing an open letter from Bonomo to Redi (16) (Figures 6.5 and 6.6).

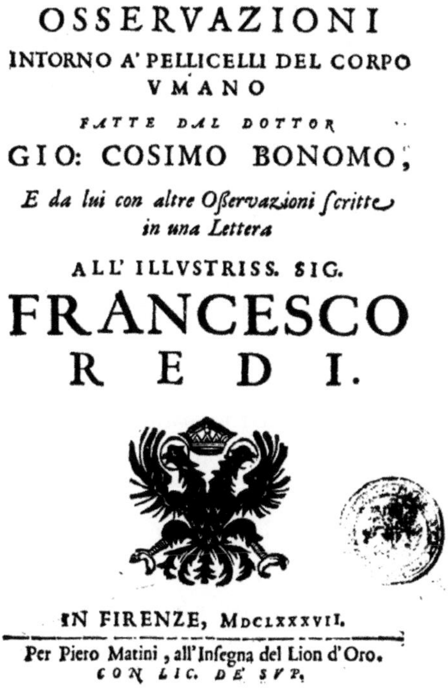

OSSERVAZIONI

INTORNO A' PELLICELLI DEL CORPO
VMANO

FATTE DAL DOTTOR

GIO: COSIMO BONOMO,

*E da lui con altre Oßervazioni fcritte
in una Lettera*

ALL' ILLVSTRISS. SIG.

**FRANCESCO
R E D I.**

IN FIRENZE, MDCLXXXVII.

Per Piero Matini , all'Infegna del Lion d'Oro.
CON LIC. DE SVP.

Figure 6.5 Bookplate of *Osservazioni intorno a' pellicelli del corpo umano*, the pamphlet where Bonomo and Cestoni first publicly declared their theory that scabies was caused by the presence of a mite in the skin.

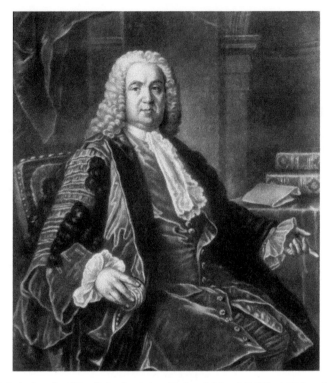

Figure 6.6 A sketch of English physician Richard Mead (1673–1754), who underwent medical training in Italy, where he came across Bonomo and Cestoni's pamphlet and submitted a translated excerpt of it to *Philosophical Transactions of the Royal Society of London* (1703), thereby introducing their theory to the English-speaking world.

The following passages are quoted verbatim from the English physician Richard Mead's 1703 abstracted translation:

Having frequently observed that the poor women when their children are troubled with The Itch, do with the point of a pin pull out of the scabby skin little bladders of water, and crack them like fleas upon their nails; and that the scabby slaves in the Bagno at Leghorne[10] do often practice this mutual kindness upon one another; it came into my mind to examine what these bladders might really be.

I quickly found an itchy person, and asking him where he felt the greatest and most acute itching, he pointed to a great many little pustules not yet scabb'd over, of which picking out one with a very fine needle, and squeezing from it a thin water, I took out a very small white globule scarcely discernible: observing this with a microscope, I found it to be a very minute living creature, in shape resembling a tortoise, of whitish colour, a little dark upon the back, with some thin and long hairs, of nimble motion, with six feet, a sharp head, with two little horns at the end of the snout ...[11]

Not satisfied with the first discovery, I repeated the search in several itchy persons of different age, complexion, and sex, and at different seasons of the year, and in all found the same animals; and that in most of the watery pustules, for now and then in some few, I could not see any.

And tho by reason of their minuteness, and colour the same with the skin, 'tis hard to discern these creatures upon the surface of the body, nevertheless I have sometimes seen them upon the joynts of the fingers in the little furrows of the cuticula, where with their sharp head they first begin to enter, and by this gnawing and working in with their body, they cause a most troublesome itching, till they are got quite under the cuticula; and then 'tis easy to see how they make ways from place to place by their biting and eating, one single one happening sometimes to make several pustules, of which I have often found two or three together, and for the most part very near to one another.

With great earnestness I examined whether or no these animalcules laid eggs, and after many enquiries, at last by good fortune while I was drawing the figure of one of 'em by a microscope, from the hinder part I saw drop a very small and scarcely visible white egg, almost transparent, and oblong, like to the seed of a pine-apple [d' un Pinocchio]...

I oftentimes found these eggs afterwards, from which no doubt these creatures are generated, as all others are, that is, from a male and female, tho I have not yet been able by any difference of figure to distinguish the sex of these animals.

From this discovery it may be no difficult matter to give a more rational account of The Itch, than authors have hitherto delivered us. It being very probable that this contagious disease owes its origin neither to the melancholy humour of Galen, nor the corrosive acid of Sylvius, nor the particular ferment of Van Helmont, not the irritating salts in the serum or lympha of the moderns, but is no other than the continual biting of these animalcules in the skin, by means of which some portion of the serum ouzing out thro the small apertures of the cutis, little watery bladders are made, within which the insects continuing to gnaw, the infected are forced to scratch, and by scratching increase the mischief, and thus renew the troublesome work, breaking not only the little pustules, but the skin too, and some little blood vessels, and to making scabs, crusty sores, and such like filthy symptoms.

From hence we come to understand how The Itch proves to be a distemper so very catching; since these creatures by simple contact can easily pass from one body to another, their motion being, wonderfully swift, and they as well crawling upon the surface of the body as under the cuticula, being very apt to stick to everything that touches 'em, and a very few of them, being once lodged, they multiply apace by the eggs which they lay.

Neither is it any wonder if this infection be propagated by the means of sheets, towels, handkerchiefs, gloves, etc. used by itchy persons; it being easy enough for some of the creepers to be lodged in such things as those; and indeed I have observed that they will live out of the body 2 or 3 days.

Nor in the last place shall we be at a loss to know the reason of the cure of this malady by lixivial washes, baths, and ointments made up with salts, sulphurs, vitriols, mercury's, simple, praecipitate or sublimate, and such sort of corrosive and penetrating medicines. These being infallibly powerful to kill the vermin lodged in the cavities of the skin; which scratching will never do, partly by reason of their hardness, and partly because they are so minute as scarcely to be found by the nails.

Neither do inward medicines perform any real service in this case, it being always necessary after a tedious use of these to have recourse to those external ones already mentioned. And if in practice we oftentimes experience, that this disease, when we think it quite cured by unction does nevertheless in a short time return again, this is not strange, since tho the oyntment may have killed all the living creatures, yet it may not probably have destroyed all their eggs, laid as it were in the nests of the skin, from which they may afterwards breed again and renew the distemper. And upon this account, 'tis very advisable after the cure is once performed, still to continue the anointing for a day or two more, which it is the easier to do, because these liniments may be agreeable enough, and of a good smell, as particularly is that compounded of the ointment of orange flowers or roses, and a small quantity of red praecipitate.[12]

As von Hebra noted nearly 150 years later, 'This pamphlet is so excellent, that even at the present day there is very little to be added to the account which it contains of scabies and the *Acarus scabiei*' (27). Bonomo and Cestoni's thorough description of the mite, linkage to the itchy skin eruption it causes, repudiation of prior erroneous theories, prescription for external treatment, and description of its method of transmissibility were seminal, farsighted, and frankly incompatible with the current state of medical knowledge. We know this specifically from the commentary of the Pope's chief physician Giovanni Maria Lancisi (1654–1720), holder of the lofty title of papal archiater (Figure 6.7).

Lancisi, a renowned physician and scientist in his own right[13] (170), was forwarded a copy of the Bonomo and Cestoni's pamphlet, as published by Redi, and found himself in the position of being the arbiter of their conclusions on scabies. Between 4 August and 15 October 1687, eight letters were exchanged between Bonomo and Lancisi, in which Bonomo advocated for his ideas and Lancisi, in his responses, at first politely and then later more bluntly dismissed Bonomo and Cestoni's work, revealing the very conservative nature of establishment medicine and science (162). These letters were later compiled by Lancisi as a manuscript entitled *Apologetic dissertation between ... GC Bonomo*

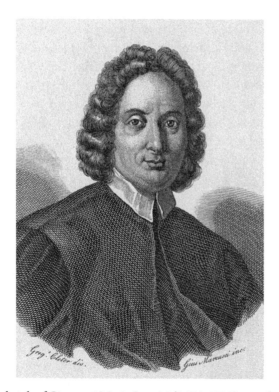

Figure 6.7 A sketch of Giovanni Maria Lancisi (1654–1720), papal archiater, who rejected Bonomo and Cestoni's theory that scabies was caused by the gnawing of a mite. Lancisi was a prominent scientist and anatomist in his own right.

and...GM Lancisi, which can now be found at the Lancisiana Library, which is located in the Santo Spirito Hospital in Rome.

A closer look at the discourse between Bonomo and Lancisi is instructive in helping to understand why *Osservazioni intorno a' pellicelli del corpo umano* did not settle the issue of the cause of scabies once and for all. Bonomo initiated the dialogue, writing to Lancisi asking him humbly to evaluate the pamphlet and submit it to the Roman Medical Congress for its consideration. Lancisi showed the pamphlet to several of his scientific colleagues, and his initial reply to Bonomo is a mixture of praise and gentle criticism. Lancisi noted that the reaction of scholars he consulted was mixed. Some were supportive of Bonomo and Cestoni's work, and Lancisi even noted one commentator knew of a woman in Rome whose sole job it was to walk around and extract mites from those affected by mange, upon which she would crush them between her fingernails eliciting a crackling noise. (Sound familiar?)

However, the majority of Lancisi's esteemed colleagues had reservations or objections to Bonomo and Cestoni's findings. For some, Bonomo's observations were dismissed as being but a product of microscopy, an illusionary tool known to deceive the senses leaving medicine and science riddled with misconception and lies. This was a not uncommon sentiment in the early days of microscopy. Here Lancisi came to Bonomo's aid, dismissing this claim as nonsense, stating that he viewed the microscope as one of the great inventions of the day.

But Lancisi rejected Bonomo and Cestoni's conclusion outright that scabies was simply due to the gnawing or biting of mites in the skin. Lancisi, who referred to Bonomo's mites as 'worms', did not doubt that Bonomo in fact had seen what he described. But to Lancisi, the supposition that these microscopic creatures could be the underlying cause of scabies and its accompanying itch was completely unfounded. Worms, Lancisi noted, could be found in a multitude of diseases, and their presence did not indicate causality. Lancisi, in spite of his achievements in science and medicine, subscribed to the long-accepted idea that scabies was fundamentally a disease of the blood. Any pustules or water blisters seen in scabies, he argued, were not due to a contagious worm, but rather (quite correctly) an aggregation of serum below the skin. And even if mites could be found in cases of scabies, this alone did not make scabies a disease attributable to an external contagious element. Aristotle's theory of spontaneous generation very straightforwardly could explain their presence. Thus when examining samples from those with scabies, the presence of minute organisms, whether they be mites, worms, or something else was a curiosity at best. To Lancisi, at least, that was the end of the matter.

Whether due to his youth or, perhaps, the courage of his convictions, Bonomo took the bold step of replying to Lancisi in rebuttal. Bonomo granted that he could not prove that all cases of scabies were due to the mites he and Cestoni had found. However, he asserted that if there were in fact other causes of scabies, they should be classified as separate diseases. Bonomo argued that because he could successfully treat all cases of scabies with external medication alone, scabies could not be a strictly internal disease. He concluded his reply by requesting Lancisi's continued support in his research endeavours, and hoping to be able to address any other doubts that Lancisi might have.

Lancisi's response to Bonomo's rebuttal, dated 20 September 1687, carries a very much changed tone from his prior letter. It comes across as a dismissive retort to a 24-year-old upstart who had directly challenged Lancisi's core knowledge. Lancisi lamented that he hoped not to have to be so blunt: why exactly did Bonomo think that after one year of study he could propose an entirely new theory of scabies that flew in the face of hundreds of years of observations by other scholars? Lancisi considered Bonomo's position pure hubris and exhorted him to consider, for a moment, that his new theory of scabies may in fact not be true. Lancisi proceeded to cite Galen, as well as more modern authors such as Fracastoro, Mercuriale, and van Helmonte, to support his traditional interpretation of scabies. Specifically with regard to Bonomo's point that topical medication would not cure scabies if it were an internal disease, Lancisi pointed out several examples to the contrary of other diseases, including skin tumours, which originate internally, but could be successfully treated with external remedies. Lancisi noted that even if some cases of scabies could be treated strictly with external preparations, it was dangerous to treat with topical remedies alone. By doing so one might suppress the healthy evacuation of fluids, perpetuate internal putrefaction, and endanger the health of the patient. Lancisi, in the fashion of a professor lecturing a pupil, further suggested Bonomo familiarize himself with a variety of passages from specific publications, or if need be, reread them.

By this stage of their correspondence, Bonomo realized that he would not be able to convince Lancisi of the validity of his theory, and thus backpedalled. Bonomo reassured Lancisi that he meant no offence, and admitted that it was possible that his eyes were playing tricks on him. He reassured that he did not wish to contradict Lancisi who had invoked the weight of history to justify his conservatism.[14] It appears that Bonomo felt more defeated and resigned rather than threatened. In ending their correspondence, Bonomo requested that Lancisi send him a high-quality microscope from Rome so that he could use it to continue his studies.

Quite remarkably, Bonomo and Cestoni's letter is arguably the first comprehensive description of an infectious organism causing disease. Some authors have gone so far as to suggest that with the publication of their pamphlet, Bonomo and Cestoni birthed the field of infectious disease and were directly responsible for toppling Galenism and ushering in a new era in medicine (56, 185).[15] In 1934, dermatologist and head of the American Medical Association, Dr William Pusey, wrote that Bonomo and Cestoni's letter constituted, 'a weighty argument against the humoral theory of skin diseases' (141). Ironically what is now viewed as landmark document, to Lancisi's eye was little more that the theories of a pushy and inexperienced young pupil. Writing on the two hundredth anniversary of Lancisi's death, Italian dermatologist Ugo Vivani blamed Lancisi for relegating Bonomo and Cestoni's ideas to the dust bin, claiming that he alone delayed the true understanding of the cause of scabies by 147 years (171), commenting resignedly: '*error humano est*'. It is not fair to lay solely blame Lancisi as his thinking was representative of entire medical establishment. The medical mind was simply not prepared for Bonomo and Cestoni's ideas. They would have to take root in a much later time, and in an entirely different place.

Yet Bonomo and Cestoni's work did not go without notice. It was translated into Latin by G. Lanzoni in 1692. The Italian educated English physician Richard Mead (1673–1754) came across their letter while travelling in Italy, and recognizing its importance, published an abstract of it, translated into English (completely omitting Redi's non-scabies-related additions), in the *Philosophical Transactions of the Royal Society of London* (1703) (18). A translation into French was published in 1757 in *Collection Academique*. And subsequently Wichmann published *Aetiologie der Krätze* in 1786 (*Etiology of Scabies*), which further disseminated the ideas of Bonomo and Cestoni, making them widely known in Germany.[16]

Meanwhile, the medical community of the seventeenth and eighteenth centuries continued to subscribe to the conviction that scabies was an internal ailment. Confusing and conflicting embellishments on this theme were common. The eminent Dutch chemist and physiologist Jan Baptiste van Helmont theorized that scabies was a cutaneous manifestation of digestive imbalance. He argued that excess stomach acid could cause 'strangury if it passes into the urine, gout if it is deposited into the joints; and scabies if it reaches the skin' (27). In 1722 Jacob Schwiebe proposed the outlandish theory that scabies derived from sweet fruits such as grapes and figs, and that 'it may either reach the skin by contact from without, or be swallowed in the fruit, in which case it is reanimated in the stomach, and creeps from that organ to other parts of the body' (27).

Moreover, the presence of a mite in lesions of scabies, as confirmed by microscopy, did not greatly trouble the medical mainstream. Its existence was dismissed as a result of the disease rather than its cause. Schubert, echoing some of Lancisi thoughts, wrote nearly a hundred years later in 1779 that:

> although I will not deny that worms really exist in the pustules of the itch, yet their presence is no proof that they are in some way or other generated by the disease; for we find worms in ulcers and wounds, and yet no one would assert that these worms give rise to the ulcers.

The theory of spontaneous generation still held broad appeal, and Redi's experiments notwithstanding, it would not be fully discarded until Louis Pasteur's nutrient broth experiments in the mid nineteenth century.

So what then was the impact of Bonomo and Cestoni's letter? Certainly it was another voice among the many that called out that the medical theories of antiquity were incomplete, at best, or frankly wrong. By the seventeenth century, the impregnability of Galen and his doctrine of the humours had come under multipronged yet disorganized attack. Many competing ideas regarding the basis of disease had been put forth and published, some incorporating Galen's humours, some invoking derivative explanations (such as 'ferments'), and others, such as iatromechanics, which were loosely based on ideas originating from Newtonian science. Physicians as a whole proved to be very traditional and largely were not a receptive audience for new ideas regarding the cause of disease. In some instances, the ability to practice medicine was only granted to those with formal education in Greek and Latin, and able to pass examinations on the theories of antiquity (140, 144). Thus findings clearly at odds with the Galenistic worldview, such as Harvey's 1628 publication demonstrating the circulation of blood, did not deal the ancient theory of humoralism the blow that in retrospect one might have imagined. And meanwhile other far-fetched explanations of disease continued to be put forth, such as those invoking the wrath of God, noxious emanations from the earth (for instance the bad air, or malaria), and even the malalignment of the celestial bodies. The term 'influenza', borrowed from Italian, specifically derives from this latter meaning—that of unfavourable astrological influences.[17] Bonomo and Cestoni's letter to Redi on the aetiology of The Itch thus came during a time of jumbled concepts, when medicine was clearly in a prolonged period of transition.

Do Bonomo and Cestoni thus deserve credit as being the persons who 'discovered' scabies? If seeing is believing, Hauptmann's 1657 sketch might arguably present the strongest claim. And others before him had written about scabies without providing a sketch. Given that for millennia largely illiterate common folk knew how to extract mites from their suffering brethren using a sewing needle, an argument can be made that it is absurd to consider any one person to be the 'discoverer' of scabies. What Bonomo and Cestoni did do was provide a thorough and comprehensive written description of The Itch. For this reason, it thus seems a fair statement to label Bonomo and Cestoni the discoverers of the acarian origin of scabies (Figure 6.8).

Specifically noteworthy was their conclusion that the explanation for The Itch was simply and directly attributable to the 'gnawing' of the scabies mite itself. Sweeping fanciful theory aside, they showed that infection could in fact have direct mechanistic underpinning. And on this topic they minced no words, explicitly dismissing different doctrines (humours, ferments, and corrosive acids) as being insufficient to account for The Itch. In the final pamphlet Redi added text touting the implications of Bonomo and Cestoni's letter. Redi

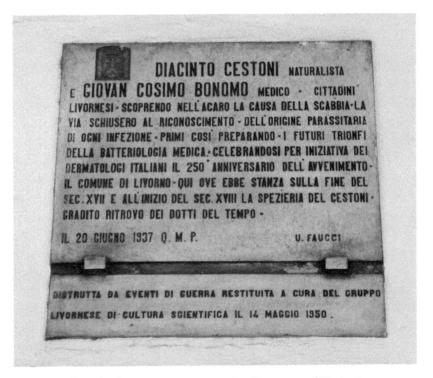

Figure 6.8 Placard in Livorno commemorating Bonomo and Cestoni.

explicitly pointed out that their findings directly contradicted the opinions of other learned men.[18]

However, it strains credibility to claim Bonomo and Cestoni overturned Galenism. Certainly their findings did not square well with the medical theories of antiquity. Their description of the acarus causing scabies provided additional evidence for animalculism. This theory, that minute animals were the cause of disease, was rapidly gaining currency with the development of microscopy, as mastered by Leeuwenhoek and others. However microscopy was in its infancy, and limited to the few who could construct and operate such devices. Broader claims that animalcules were responsible for a host of infectious diseases including whooping cough, syphilis, and dysentery (described by the English physician John Nyander as 'an internal itch of the intestines') (165) could not be reliably supported by microscopic observations, leading many to dismiss animalculism outright (144). Moreover positive microscopic findings which appeared to fly in the face of common experience led many (205), including associates of Lancisi, to regard microscopy with great suspicion. Add to this that Bonomo incorrectly described where the mite resided (pustule), and thus for a multitude of reasons, Bonomo and Cestoni's findings were not readily appreciated or easily replicated.[19]

The medical mainstream was thus not appreciably influenced by the publication of *Osservazioni intorno a' pellicelli del corpo umano*. Even an enlightened physician like Mead seems not to have been overly influenced by Bonomo and Cestoni's findings, as his later writing on the plague showed that he continued to rely on Galenic humours, at least in part, in his discussion of disease.[20] In spite of this, there is some evidence, however, that their ideas were circulated. In 1722 the Vice-President of the Royal Society, Hans Sloane, suggested that the microscopic studies of Bonomo and Cestoni should be additionally investigated, and extended to other diseases to determine if similarly one could, 'observe, whether any insects are to be found in ye pustules of those that are ill of ye small pox' (140). Yet for the most part, Bonomo and Cestoni's work came to a temporary dead end.

Because of the very conservative nature of medicine and the men who practiced it,[21] it thus fell upon those professions at the periphery of medicine to make incremental progress. The Swedish naturalist Carl Linnaeus recognized the existence of the itch mite, and in his 1746 *Fauna Swezica*, issued it a formal classification: *Acarus humanus-subcutaneus*. In doing so, he officially recognized scabies as being an eight-legged arachnid formally not belonging to same category as the six-legged insect.[22] Veterinarians demonstrated the presence of morphologically similar itch mites on other species, and showed their contagiousness through experimentation (152). Naturalists and entomologists, such as Charles deGeer in 1778, published some of the earliest accurate drawings of *Sarcoptes scabiei*, and that made it increasingly difficult to deny its existence if not its import. The French entomologist Latreille established the genus Sarcoptes and named the scabies mite *Sarcoptes scabiei*, derived from the Greek and meaning 'flesh cutter'. Yet Renaissance medicine continued to be largely unmoved, as von Hebra pointed out:

> The great authorities in dermatology at the time cared very little for the labours of men of science; and the majority of medical practitioners were in the habit of relying upon the statements of those who were at the head of their profession, without making any independent inquiries of their own.

Nearly 100 years after Bonomo and Cestoni's reports, in 1786, the German physician Johann Wichmann published *Etiology of Scabies* (*Aetiologie der Krätze*) in Hannover. In this work, he brilliantly summarized the current state of knowledge, and emphasized the parasitic nature of scabies, thrusting the topic back into the public sphere after a long period of dormancy. According to von Hebra, Wichmann 'did more than all others to make generally known the mite-theory of scabies.' In the second edition of *Etiology of Scabies*, published in 1791, Wichmann described the first account of the experimental transmissibility of scabies by demonstrating that scabies could be transferred to a person who had voluntarily infected himself with an adult female mite. Yet even this eye-opening piece of information was largely ignored. Ironically, anyone looking to understand scabies would have done best simply by consulting the dictionary (150). The entry for 'itch' in Dr Samuel Johnson's Dictionary (1755), reveals a sophisticated general understanding. Here 'itch' was defined as a 'cutaneous disease extremely contagious which overspreads the body with small pustules filled with thin serum, and raised, as microscopes have discovered, by a small animal. It is cured by sulphur.' (20)

For years after Bonomo and Cestoni's publication, peasant and village elders continued to remain the best source for practical knowledge on The Itch. In 1801 the physician Joseph Adams recounted a demonstration, on the Portuguese island of Madeira, in which an old villager woman showed him how to find the itch mite, which the locals called 'an ouçao' (136):

> In searching for the insect, in which was regularly instructed by the old lady before mentioned, the bladder (vesicle) is always passed over, if a red and, as it appears by the microscope, a somewhat knotty line is discovered to issue

from it; at the end of this line, which is about a quarter of an inch long, is found a reddish elevation, to appearance dry and firm. Under this parts of the ouçao are sometimes discoverable with a good glass, but whether this is the case or not, this is the only place in which the ouçao is expected and if not found here, the search is abandoned.

In this passage, Adams relates that the layperson knew exactly where to look for the mite—at the end of the burrow not in the surrounding blister.[23] Adams advanced his understanding a step further, having mites extracted from a young girl and affixed to the fingers of his left hand. He wrote:

For more than three weeks (thereafter) little or no inconvenience was felt. From that time began frequent itching in different parts of my body and arms, but no eruption could be discovered. In less than a fortnight afterward, my arms and belly were covered with a general efflorescence, but few vesicles appeared. I applied to my old woman, who readily drew two ouçöes from my arm.

In addition to successfully transferring scabies to himself, Adams proceeded to inadvertently spread it to several members of his family. By isolating a scabies mite from a diseased individual, using this mite to infect himself with scabies, and then reisolating a mite from his lesions, Adams had, without realizing it, formally satisfied Koch's postulates, a set of rules later formulated by the bacteriologist Robert Koch used to prove that an agent causes an infectious disease (123). Adams thus found himself in a position to crown himself the modern day discoverer of scabies. In the end, however, he failed to connect the dots and concluded that The Itch and the illness caused by ouçöes were in fact two distinct diseases. Yet another opportunity had been lost to reveal the true cause of scabies. But within a generation, the Corsican medical student Simon François Renucci would put the issue to rest in nineteenth-century Paris, the medical centre of the world in its day.

Notes

1. Elsewhere, in describing creatures that generate from wood and wax, Aristotle described the 'smallest of animalcules' as a mite or 'akari', an animal so minute as to be indivisible. Again, from the passage it is somewhat obscure exactly what he was referring to. Irrespective, nearly 2000 years later, European observers would borrow his terminology to name the causative mite of scabies, labelling it as *Acarus scabiei*.

2. Early written mention of lay knowledge can be found in the writings of the sixteenth-century French physician Guilaumme Rondelet: 'Women extract them with a needle and so relieve themselves of the itching' (125).

3. Today such wisdom is often derided as being old-wives tales.

4. For example, al-Tabari's description of papulo-pustular scabies is as follows:
   > Papulo-pustular scabies: characterized by large, disseminated papules, the bases of which are hard and elevated above the level of the skin. Pus fills the upper third or upper half of the papule and in the latter instance one can differentiate two equal parts of the papule, the upper full of pus, the lower red and hard. When the pus is gone, the lower part remains as a smooth cone-like elevation, from the surface of which, a yellow water oozes. This type itches little. The cause is thick, black-bile-like mixture, which is brought about through decay and decomposition through moisture.

   Today we might recognize this condition as impetigo, or a superficial bacterial infection. It is also possible that al-Tabari here is describing cases of infected scabies. His reference to bodily humours shows that his general medical knowledge very much fit in to the Galenist paradigm of the day.

5. *'Et se'el n'a mains beles et netes /Ou de sirons, ou du bubetes /Gart que lessier ne les i vueille /Face les oster a l'agueille /Ou ses mains en ses gans repoigne'*

6. In my personal experience, patients with scabies today seldomly have pustules. Likely this is due to modern standards of personal hygiene as well as the availability of effective antimicrobial agents.

7. Wichmann writes that those looking in the pustule contents would be let down as they, 'expect to find a large worm visible to the naked eye as each pustule is opened' (124).

8. Bonomo and Cestoni's original letter was only rediscovered in 1925 by Alberto Razzauti, which was lying preserved amongst an indexed collection of Redi's papers held in the library of Fraternita di S. Maria of Arezzo. The historical document is not without controversy, however. Towards the end of his life, in 1710, Cestoni wrote to fellow Italian naturalist Sig. Antonio Vallisnieri stating that, 'The observations concerning the flesh-worms of the human body which, in 1687, appeared in Florence under the name of D. Gio. Cosimo Bonomo in a letter to Sig. Francesco Redi, were all of them my discoveries, the results of my repeated and very assiduous experiments.' Likely Cestoni felt frustrated that many attributions made left his name out. For reasons unclear, the original letter was published with the title *Osservazioni intorno a' pellicelli del corpo umano fatte dal dottor Gio. Cosimo Bonomo ... a illustriss Sig. Francesco Redi*, leaving out Cestoni's name from the title altogether. The text of the letter does indeed refer to Cestoni and his vast experience. However, Mead's communication to the Royal Society in London followed suit and was entitled 'An abstract of a letter from Dr. Bonomo to Signior Redi', introducing the finding into the English literature as if they were Bonomo's alone.

   The story might stop there; however, the eminent nineteenth-century French dermatologist Raspail, who will be encountered later in our narrative, interpreted this to signify that Bonomo did not in fact exist and was but the pen-name that Cestoni assumed under which to publish his controversial ideas. Subsequent authors adopted this viewpoint citing Raspail. However other eminent authors such as Furstenberg rejected this claim. In a 1949 monograph, Dr Friedman carefully examined these claims drawing on Italian sources, and rejected the notion that Bonomo was not a real person or was not involved in the discovery (147). Razzauti also discredited Cestoni's 1710 claim that he was the true discoverer of the acarian origin of scabies, dismissing it as 'senile vanity' (147).

9. Ironically in his letter to Redi, Bonomo and Cestoni complained about the quality of their microscope, calling it *'povero e debole microscopio'* or a 'poor and weak microscope'. They petitioned to Rome to send better equipment.

10. Reference to the bathhouses at Livorno.

11. If in fact the mite that Bonomo describes had six legs (feet), it would be an immature mite form. Dr Meinking, Taplin, and Vicaria propose that Bonomo, 'confuse[d] the two pediculate suckers on the anterior legs as horns, and [thus] ... he did in fact retrieve an eight-legged adult *Sarcoptes scabiei'* (151).

12. In 1937 the unabridged text of Bonomo's original letter to Redi was published by Friedman (166) (translated into English with the assistance of Messrs E. Antonelli, O.A. Mirarchi, and F. Baccari). By comparing Bonomo and Cestoni's original letter with Redi's published pamphlet, one can see specific additions that Redi made. For example the language describing the scabies mite as 'resembling a tortoise' is nowhere to be found in the original letter. Moreover one can also appreciate liberties that Mead took in translation. For instance Bonomo describes scabies eggs as resembling 'un Pinocchio', which might be more aptly translated as a 'pine nut' rather than Mead's 'seed of a pine-apple'. Nevertheless Redi's modifications of Bonomo and Cestoni's original letter, as printed in *Osservazioni intorno a' pellicelli del corpo umano*, and Mead's abstracted 1703 translation of it would have been what were available to the Italian and English speaking public, respectively.

13. Lancisi's formidable medical achievements included advances in neuroanatomy and cardiac anatomy, the description of a link between sudden death and myocardial disease, an early classification of aneurysms, a description of the pathological mechanism of urine formation, and an early description of the corpus callosum. His 1717 publication *De noxiis paludum effluviis* supported the miasmatic aetiology of malaria, thus also making him one of the leading epidemiological thinkers of his days. He advocated draining swampland as a preventative measure against malaria (170).

14. Or, as Bonomo wrote, *'tanto piu che mi fa conoscere, che fino la storia sacra mi peruade il contrario.'*

15. Friedman proposed that 20 June 1937, the 250th anniversary of Bonomo's letter to Redi, be pronounced 'Scabies Day', in recognition of 'the establishment, for the first time in the history of medicine, of a specific cause for any of the diseases known to man, and hence constitutes the first concrete example of the theory of specificity in the etiology of disease'. He additionally noted it was a day worth commemorating 'because it definitely marks the beginning of the end of the Doctrine of Humoralism, which, as a pathological concept, had dominated medicine since the time of Hippocrates and Galen' (164).

16. In 1936 Friedman published a partial English translation of Wichmann's seminal work with contemporaneous as well and more modern commentary (124).

17. The alignment of the celestial bodies helped explain why certain diseases of contagion might be more limited in nature, whereas others erupted into devastating pandemics. The configuration of Mars with respect to Saturn was thought to be potentially very important in this regard (168).

18. Redi added:

> *or tra tante opinioni qual misfatto mai mi sarebbe, fe ancor io andaffi opinando diversamente da questi dottissimi Vomini? O per ischerzo che si sia, o, pure, com'e piu facile, per da vero, Io per ora mi sento inclinato a voler credere, che la Rogna, da Latini chiatmata scabies, e descritta per un male cutaneo, ed appiccaticcio, no fia altro, che una morficatura, o rosicatura pruringinosa, e continua fattanella cute de' nostri corpi da questi soprammentovati Bacolini.*

The English translation is, roughly:

> Between all of these wrong opinions, how would I look if I went against all these other well educated men? Whether it is a joke or reality, at this moment, I feel inclined to believe that mange, whom the Latins called scabies is nothing more than a contagious skin disease, caused by the bite of a little animal called Bacolini whose incessant gnawing of the skin causes intense itchiness.

19. In 1688, however, the priest, physician, and philosopher Carolus Musitanus would rectify Bonomo and Cestoni's error, describing the exact location of the scabies mite in the burrow (175):

> [The mites] crawl under the skin, from one place to another, making burrows, in the manner of moles, and frequently long ones, as though they were dragging ploughs behind them. At the same time they produce a very annoying itching. Thus they creep about under the skin and can be readily observed as they migrate from one place of abode to another. Furthermore, if you wish, you might be able, with the point of a pin, to pluck the animalcule out from the end of the burrow.

With this last essential piece of information by Musitanus, by the late seventeenth century, all the clues to fully understanding the nature of scabies were available. However Musitanus' work was not widely read. It would take an additional 150 years for the medical community to come around to fully accepting the itch mite as the cause of scabies.

20. In Mead's 1720 treatise on the plague, *A Short Discourse Concerning Pestilential Contagion and Those Methods to be Used to Prevent It*, he put forth many practical suggestions for dealing with the plague, such as burying the dead deep in the earth away from where people live. However he also suggested putting 'the humours of the body into such as state as to not be alterable by the matter of infection', such as by, 'living with temperance upon a good generous diet and avoiding fastings, watchings, and extreme weariness, etc ... ' (142). Thus more than 15 years after publishing Bonomo and Cestoni's letter in English, he was still, at least in some part, subscribing to Galenistic concepts.

21. Friedman gives an idea how ingrained Galenic principles were, writing:

> True, so venerated and powerful was the word of Authority, so universal was its acceptance, so fearful were physicians of questioning the infallibility of Galenic dogma, and so severe was the punishment meted out on occasion by the Faculties (particularly the Paris Faculty of the Seventeenth Century), to any who dared be guilty of heretical inclinations, that brave and fearless indeed had to be he who dared investigate for himself and, perhaps, raise his voice in disaffirmation or denial of orthodox teachings. (125)

22. Linnaeus firmly believed in animate pathogenesis and animalculism. That The Itch was well-known to be caused by a mite burrowing in the skin was used to buttress his arguments. However when others were unable to find the scabies mite, either due to the poor

quality of their instrumentation or searching for the mite in the wrong place (pustules), the tendency was to discredit animalculism as a whole. Thus in some instances the rudimentary science of microscopy actually retarded progress.

23. Adams pointed out that knowledge of the itch mite was far more advanced among commoners than physicians:

> By this time the reader will be convinced, that to find the names of this insect in different languages, he must look to the dictionaries; and to learn how to find the insect itself, he must consult nurses, or those who are ready to learn the habits of every class. (136)

7

Early Pioneers

Alibert and Renucci

The medical establishment only very belatedly came to accept that scabies is directly caused by the itch mite, *Sarcoptes scabiei*. The denouement of our story takes place at the Hôpital Saint-Louis in Paris. Built on the outskirts of town in 1607 as a plague hospital (which today leaves it lying in the middle of the 10th arrondissement), it served as focal point for the treatment of the Parisian pandemic of the day. At various times it housed those suffering from the plaque, cholera, smallpox, typhus, scurvy, and syphilis, as well as ulcerative skin diseases, which regardless of cause, were confusingly and reflexively lumped together (139).[1] By the late eighteenth century, increasing urbanization and crowding in the capital led to a dramatic increase in the number of scabies cases in Paris. A localized centre was needed to treat these contagious cases. The Hôpital Saint-Louis fit the bill (Figure 7.1).

Scabies patients from other hospitals were specifically sent there, and new cases quickly filled the wards. By the beginning of the nineteenth century, the Hôpital Saint-Louis routinely housed hundreds of patients suffering from The Itch. Under its director Jean-Louis Alibert (1768–1837), the Hôpital developed into a leading specialized centre for the treatment of skin disease (Figure 7.2).

Interestingly Alibert, widely considered to be the father of modern French dermatology, began his career, studying for the seminary. His education, however, was truncated due to the closing of religious orders that occurred during the French Revolution. He subsequently matriculated at the Paris Medical School in 1796, where he performed well in botany, obstetrics, and internal pathology, but ironically only obtained weak marks in external pathology (159)! Alibert was appointed physician to the Hôpital Saint-Louis in 1802, where he intensely observed all kinds of patients who suffered from a wide variety of skin maladies. With this material, he quickly developed a mastery of skin disease. Moreover, he developed a reputation for being kind, courteous, and caring. When travelling in his carriage, if he saw someone with an unusual or severe skin manifestation, he would stop and take them to the Hôpital

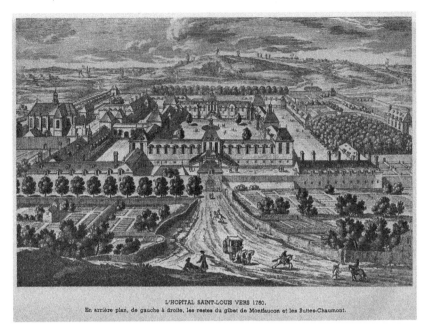

L'HOPITAL SAINT-LOUIS VERS 1760.
En arrière plan, de gauche à droite, les restes du gibet de Montfaucon et les Buttes-Chaumont.

Figure 7.1 A sketch of Hôpital Saint-Louis in Paris. Originally built on the outskirts of the city as a plaque hospital, by the eighteenth century, it had become a clearinghouse for scabies cases.

for treatment. The reputation of the Hôpital was such that it drew severe skin cases not just from Paris, or even France, but from Europe as a whole, leaving even Alibert in amazement, proclaiming it 'the sewer of all the countries of the world' (161). In short, the breadth and depth of skin pathology to be seen at the Hôpital was unmatched by any other institution at the time.

Aside from being a renowned physician and dermatologist,[2] Alibert was also a great teacher drawing pupils from across France and the rest of Europe. His lectures were so well attended they caused the amphitheatre to overflow and had to be moved outdoors. On the hospital grounds, he would stand next to his patients, who had hung on their chest a placard with the title of their disorder, and lecture on their condition (160). He summarized his clinical expertise in book entitled *A Description of the Diseases of the Skin Observed at the Hôpital Saint-Louis and an Exposition of the Best Methods Followed in Their Treatment*. Prior to the advent of photography, he had this text ornately illustrated making it the original atlas of dermatology. Alibert chose to write in the French vernacular rather than Latin, and spent a considerable sum of his own money to get his work illustrated and published.

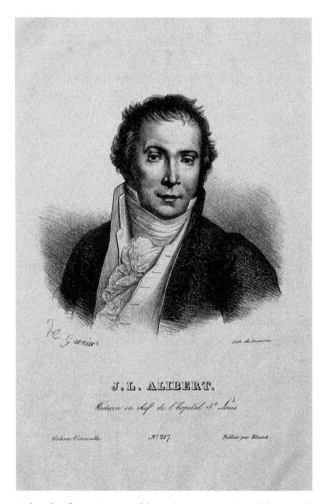

Figure 7.2 A sketch of Jean-Louis Alibert (1768–1837), widely considered to be the father of the French school of dermatology.

Alibert disparaged humoralism, and was an adherent and proponent of animalculism. Though he lacked proof, Alibert suspected that scabies was caused by a mite. He maintained this position in his lectures and teaching, which in some quarters drew great ridicule. Alibert appears to have been aware of Bonomo and Cestoni's famous letter to Redi (139), as well as the work of naturalists who had studied the scabies mite. He had tried and failed, however, to transmit scabies by inoculating the pus of scabietic lesions into others.

Thus in the year 1812, when one of his pupils, the pharmacist Jean Chrysanthe Galès, was looking for a subject for his graduation thesis, Alibert encouraged him to study scabies. Alibert, renowned for his sense of humour, reportedly said 'Compose your thesis on scabies, your name gives you the right' ('gale' being the French word for 'scabies') (129).[3] Using a good microscope, Galès reported that he was able to find mites on many, though not all patients afflicted with scabies. Over the course of 3 months of his studies, Galès recorded finding over 300 mites by examining the pustules of infested individuals. He noted several distinct species of the itch mite, which differed from one another. Galès appeared to have observed not only the itch mite, *Sarcoptes scabiei,* but also the flour mite *Acarus siro.* He performed inoculation experiments with these various mites, and described that only one kind, presumably *Sarcoptes scabiei,* could cause The Itch (139). He had a figure of the mite engraved by a medical artist—however, it appears that what was ultimately illustrated was in fact the flour or cheese mite.[4]

As it turns out, Galès like many others before him erroneously thought that the scabies mite resided in the pustule proper. Thus other physicians searching the pustules of similarly afflicted patients could not reproduce his work and routinely came away empty handed, casting doubt on the 'insect hypothesis'.[5] While a few authors such as Moffet and Musitanus had in fact described the true location of the mite (at the end of the burrow), even farsighted thinkers such as Bonomo and Cestoni had been confused on this point. That Galès misidentified the location of the mite should thus come as no surprise. The fact that he was still able to find so many mites is perhaps what is more puzzling.

Alibert was encouraged by Galès findings, but other prominent colleague physicians remained sceptical and unconvinced. Slowly the faculty divided along lines of those who believed that scabies was caused by a mite, and those who didn't. This latter group, the antiacarian camp, generated a number of reasons why scabies was not a mite disease. Likely their resistance was a combination of inherent conservatism and allegiance to dogma, though scientific scepticism certainly played a part.[6] In true academic fashion, a heated and acrimonious debate erupted. In a sense this was more than just a debate about the cause of The Itch; rather two very different paradigms of disease were battling each other. Passions flared, and in the end, a challenge was issued. In 1829, Alibert's student Jean Lugol offered a prize of 300 French francs to the individual who could prove the existence of the scabies mite.[7]

The physician François Vincent Raspail took up the challenge but, after searching through hundreds of pustules, was unable to demonstrate a single mite.[8] Then deviously turning to trickery, and to discredit Galès, he set up a public demonstration on 3 September 1829. Here, he examined a pustule from a patient with scabies and was able to demonstrate the presence of a small mite in front of a crowd of observers. The mite bore great resemblance to Galès' engraving. However Raspail immediately confessed that he had played a trick on the crowd and that his finding was nothing more than a cheese mite that had been snuck in by an accomplice.

The pro-acarian faction moved to parry and counterattack, but repeated attempts to demonstrate the presence of the itch mite in patients were unsuccessful. In spite of the fact that the scabies mite had been detected by many over the past centuries, the pro-acarian school could not locate the mite, for, as we know, they were searching in the wrong place—the vesicle or blister, rather than the end of burrow.[9]

Finally, the issue was put to rest in 1834 by the young Corsican medical student, Simon François Renucci. Like Bonomo and Cestoni, Renucci had previously witnessed village women from his home in Corsica extracting the mite with a needle from afflicted children. On multiple occasions he had extracted the mite himself. He knew from experience that the mite was to be found at the end of the burrow and not in the vesicle or pustule. When Renucci became aware of the scabies controversy raging through the Parisian faculty, he chose to interject himself into the debate. But first, just to be sure that this was in fact the same disease he knew from back home, he examined several scabietic patients in Paris and confirmed that he again could isolate mites from their skin. Knowing exactly where to find the mite, he arranged a public demonstration in which he showed off his skill. On 13 August 1834, repeatedly and on multiple attempts, Renucci was able to isolate a mite from the hands of a young woman covered in pustules in front of an audience of fellow Parisian medical students (Figure 7.3). He did the same successfully on an another, a male patient. In each instance he placed the extracted mite on his fingernail for onlookers to examine under direct sunlight from all angles. Subsequently it was examined under the microscope. Soon after, on 25 August 1834, he repeated the feat in the presence of a large number of distinguished physicians and scientists. Further sessions were performed for the benefit of sceptics including Raspail. Later in the year, he would describe his findings in his thesis titled: *On the Discovery of the Insect Which Produces the Contagion of Itch, Prurigo, and Phlyzacia*, in which he wrote:

Whenever these white or brownish points are visible at the end of the burrow they are a certain index of the presence of the Acarus. When such a point has been found, the epidermis is pierced with either a pin or a needle, half a line from the white point, towards which the pin or the needle should always be directed. One should not pierce too deeply or the mite will be injured.

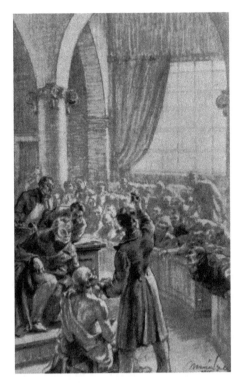

Figure 7.3 A charcoal depiction of Simon François Renucci (1794–1884) demonstrating the presence of the scabies mite in skin lesions to a faculty of onlookers in Paris. Sketched by Gyula (Jules) Merész Müller (1888–1949).
Reproduced from Nékam, Lajos A. (1936). *De Dermatologia et Dermatologis*. Budapestini.

The point of the pin or needle should be passed underneath the white point and the Acarus lifted up. It appears to have its head within a shell much like a tortoise. It is of the utmost importance to search for and locate the white point, which has not been mentioned by any other author. In human itch, the Acarus is never found in the content of the vesicles.

In accordance with the rapidly changing times, the medical community finally appeared ready to concede. Lugol graciously conceded and Renucci humbly collected his reward of 300 francs. Alibert died 3 short years later, having seen his hypothesis finally proven and the itch mite, *Sarcoptes scabiei*, accepted as the cause of scabies.[10] In addition, the first demonstration of an infectious disease had concluded. Renucci found himself in the right place at the right time (Figure 7.4).

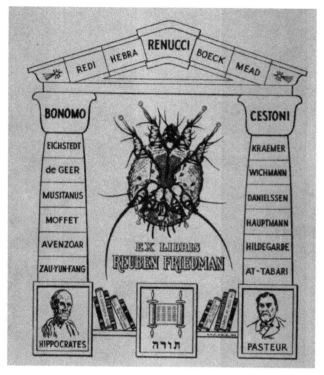

Figure 7.4 Bookplate of Reuben Friedman, twentieth-century scholar of scabies. The main contributors in the history of scabies are represented. Renucci is the keystone.
Courtesy of the owner.

Through observation, skill, sheer luck, and the courage to take the academic establishment head on, he earned himself a place in history as the modern day discoverer of scabies. By 'proving' that scabies is caused by a mite, he arguably formally described the first infectious disease. The discovery of other infectious diseases rapidly followed. In 1839, the German physician Johann Lucas Schönlein (1793–1864) discovered that the skin illness called favus was in fact due to the presence of a fungus. Shortly after fungi were additionally isolated from thrush and ringworm. A veritable explosion of discoveries of organisms (or 'animalcules') causing infectious diseases had begun.

Without a doubt, the discovery of the aetiology of scabies was an important landmark in the development of our understanding of infectious disease. Early proponents of the communicability of disease routinely listed scabies amongst those diseases that could be spread from person to person. The knowledge that The Itch had a definable cause likely provided inspiration for physicians and scientists to consider that other communicable diseases such as the plaque, yellow fever, smallpox, typhus, and cholera might have a definable causes as well.[11] Yet, because of the minute nature of their corresponding pathogens, simple microscopic investigation would be insufficient to elucidate them. Decades of addition research involving detailed epidemiological investigation would be needed to define their mechanism of contagion, and then ultimately sophisticated microbiological studies would be required to define them.

The discovery of the aetiology of scabies took place in a period characterized by opposing intellectual forces and by the divorce of science from theology and philosophy (56). As von Hebra wrote in the time leading up to the 'rediscovery' of scabies:

> If medical men in those days had but observed with unprejudiced eyes the fa-vorable results which followed the use of popular remedies and cures for sca-bies, they probably would have sooner acquired correct notions concerning the nature and treatment of the disease. But more importance was then at-tached to theoretical pedantry that to the observation of the facts ...

The antiacarian camp held on for at least a decade claiming that the Acarus, while found in scabies, was incidental and not its underlying cause. They did not concede until the publication of von Hebra's landmark treatise on scabies in 1844, and stragglers, amongst whom could be counted eminent dermatolo-gists, would hold out for yet another generation.

von Hebra

For much of history, scabies and 'The Itch' had been used loosely to denote a wide variety of often itchy rashes, whose origin was poorly understood at best. It is only over the last 2 centuries that terms describing these rashes narrowed in scope to specifically signify the itchy communicable skin disease cause by the mite *Sarcoptes scabiei*. This was largely due to the pioneering efforts of one man, the renowned physician Ferdinand Ritter von Hebra (Figure 7.5).

Through his insights, writings, and teachings, he became the dominant force that catapulted scabies into the modern era. von Hebra was instrumental in de-fining the true nature of scabies. If later Mellanby was able to see farther, it was by standing on von Hebra's shoulders.

von Hebra (1816–1880) emerged from humble beginnings, but by the end of his career, he could arguably be called the father of modern day dermatology.

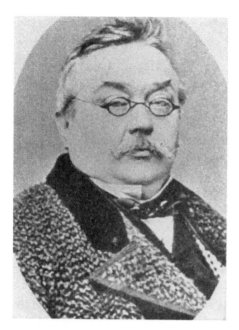

Figure 7.5 A photo of Ferdinand Ritter von Hebra (1816–1880), who mastered the topic of scabies and spread his knowledge worldwide through his pupils. Considered by many to be greatest dermatologist of his day.

The son of a quartermaster, von Hebra was born in the Austro-Hungarian town of Brno.[12] He undertook medical training in Vienna. In the early 1840's, he apprenticed with the famous physician Joseph Skoda, an early pioneer in clinical investigation, and head of the department of chest diseases. At the time, skin disease as a field of study was largely ignored and subject to general disdain given its association with venereal and other communicable disease such as leprosy. In mid-nineteenth-century Vienna, patients with chronic skin disorders too gruesome to be tolerated by polite society, including syphilitics suffering from neurological symptoms, were reflexively lumped together and treated in an annex of Skoda's chest clinic called 'the scabies station', an arrangement that seems bizarre by today's standards (80). The use of the term 'scabies' to nonspecifically lump together a variety of severe and chronic skin ailments belied the poor general state of knowledge regarding scabies, and skin disease in general (138), even in an advanced academic arena such as Vienna.[13]

In fact, the use of the term 'scabies' to designate a multitude of overlapping skin disorders dated back for hundreds of years,[14] though ironically for much of this time knowledge existed that scabies was in fact caused by a small mite. As has been mentioned, this was particularly true among the peasant class, whose view of life was uncomplicated by the medical theories of antiquity (124). Even at the time of Skoda's 'scabies station', at least a decade had passed since the formal academic demonstration in Paris, the hub of continental medicine, that mites were present in the lesions of scabies. Time would be required for this knowledge to disseminate and antiquated dogma to yield.

Skoda was a master of clinical observation and made many contributions to medicine including advances in auscultation, the art of using the stethoscope to examine the heart and lungs (109). Recognizing the rudimentary state of knowledge with regard to skin disorders in 'the scabies station', Skoda decided to recruit a colleague to help in this area. Noting von Hebra's overall high aptitude coupled with his interest in the skin, Skoda suggested that von Hebra concern himself primarily with disorders of this neglected organ system. What to others might have been perceived as a demotion, von Hebra embraced. He familiarized himself thoroughly with the state of the field, began to lecture on dermatology, and assumed charge of the dermatology clinic in the Wiener Allgemeines Krankenhaus where before long he attracted widespread recognition for his attention to detail and mastery of the subject. Within a short period of time, von Hebra gained a reputation and a following, establishing the Viennese school as the leading centre of dermatology, even surpassing the Hôpital St. Louis in Paris. Pupils would make the pilgrimage to von Hebra's clinic from throughout Europe and even the United States to learn from the master.

von Hebra was familiar with the recent breakthrough demonstrations in Paris showing that a mite could repeatedly be isolated from the skin lesions of scabies. He thus set about to understand more fully the role of the scabies mite in The Itch by studying those in the 'scabies station' who had veritable scabies. To further advance his understanding, he performed a series of self-inoculation experiments, 'that bordered on the masochistic' (24). After a period of intense study, he published his treatise on scabies in 1844. His writings were so masterly and compelling that readers were left with no doubt that the cause of scabies was a tiny mite. Amongst his many contributions, von Hebra correctly described that scabies was strictly a skin disease and not a cutaneous manifestation of any other internal disease. He clearly communicated that the presence of the burrow was the unique clinical characteristic of scabies. He was the first to describe that the widespread rash and itching of scabies was due to a person's reaction ('irritation') to the mite. In addition, he eschewed oral therapies for scabies insisting on topical treatment alone. von Hebra even performed experiments showing that topical therapy directly killed mites and cured scabies, rather than having indirect action through absorption into the bloodstream (27).

In the history of scabies, von Hebra and his treatise represent the inflection point where scabies as a disease was transformed from a collection of non-specific skin ailments to a particular pathological process, albeit with protean manifestations, caused by the itch mite *Sarcoptes scabiei*.[15] Over the course of his career, von Hebra observed over 40,000 cases of scabies, and from this wealth of clinical exposure was able to draw many astute conclusions. He noted the intensity of the itch that scabies caused is severe and suggested that only those who had actually suffered from it could understand its magnitude. His description of the diverse manifestations of skin lesions seen in scabies set the standard for all modern texts that have since followed. It behoves even experienced physicians today to go back and read von Hebra's writings on scabies as they contain a wealth of practical information.[16] von Hebra started his observations with the understated, but obvious: the earliest manifestation of scratching in scabies is four parallel red lines each corresponding to the size of the fingernail, and each separated from its neighbour by a finger's width. Repetitive scratching blurs this pattern and produces an overall general redness, and in some, individual wheals or hives can form. von Hebra proceeded to describe that additional scratching leads to epidermal disruption which thereby permits the formation of a variety of lesions of varied appearance. von Hebra thus implied that the lesions of scabies would frustrate the strict dermatological taxonomist as they do not fit neatly into one simple reaction pattern or morphology. Hence most any rash, under the right circumstances, could in fact be scabies. But far from being caused by foul humours trying to escape the body, von Hebra in no uncertain terms described that the wide variety and distribution of lesions in scabies were caused by nothing more than scabies itself or the body's reaction to the mite.

Over the course of his illustrious and prolific career von Hebra established himself as a world authority on skin disease.[17] Aside from his work on scabies, he additionally described and characterized several other skin disorders for the first time. His influence cannot be overstated. von Hebra was instrumental in defining the field of dermatology, in which the skin is recognized as an organ of study in its own right rather than simply a site which could manifest signs of internal disease. His work on scabies was and remains classic nearly 200 years after the fact. In one fell swoop he lifted the medical profession out of its confusion and rendered clarity on the subject of scabies. Within his lifetime, his students and pupils would transmit his learnings far and wide.[18]

Notes

1. Skin ulcers continue to be a source of common confusion for practicing dermatologists to this day.
2. Amongst others, Alibert was the first to recognize and describe many skin conditions including mycosis fungoides, keloids, acromegaly, and scleroderma. He coined the term 'syphilid' (159).
3. '*Composez-la sur la gale, vouz y avez des droits par votre nom*' (123) or '*composez votre these sur la gale, votre nom vous permet d'y pretender*' (163).
4. In the second half of the pamphlet *Osservazioni intorno a' pellicelli del corpo umano*, Redi added content on the cheese mite that was not present in Bonomo's original letter. Redi noted that the those who make cheese describe a certain 'cheese powder' which they consider a kind of dust, but which in fact is a great concentration of cheese mites.
5. In 1828, their *Treatise on Diseases of the Skin*, Cazenave and Schedel wrote:
   as to the proximate cause of scabies, it is still unknown. It has been in turn attributed to an acid principle, to a special ferment, and finally, the presence of an insect. This last hypothesis is still held by a great number of physicians. However, if we cannot affirm that it does not exist at all, at least we are very far from believing it. Until Galès again shows it to us, we believe ourselves justified in holding that the acarus does not exist. (123)
6. As Wichmann pointed out, 'In the science of medicine, doubt is a more pardonable sin than superstition' (124).
7. Lugol had previously performed inoculation experiments to demonstrate the contagiousness of the pustule contents in scabies. He inoculated himself, 12 students, a nurse, and 'a sister of charity' on the fingers, backs of hand, and inner wrist, areas the mite was known to favour. None of those inoculated contracted scabies. To Lugol this signified that no mite existed in scabies (17).
8. Raspail proceeded to have a long and distinguished career in science and politics. Boulevard Raspail in Paris is named in his honour.
9. The burrow was only formally described by Karl Ferdinand Eichstedt in 1846.
10. The best readily available account, in English, of the historical events surrounding Renucci's demonstration can be found in *The Dermatology and Syphilology of the Nineteenth Century* by J. Crissey and L. Parish (129).
11. The English physician William Budd (1811–1880) wrote of his confidence that typhoid fever was spread by an agent in patients' diarrheal discharge, 'as being as sure as that itch is contagious, and that smallpox may be inoculated'.
12. Brno also happens to be where the monk Gregor Mendel undertook his groundbreaking studies on pea crossing, ultimately birthing the field of genetics.
13. Just as scabies had been a term lacking precision, 'The Itch' had historically been used in a pejorative and not altogether specific sense lumping together those suffering from scabies with multiple otherwise equally disparaged diseases including leprosy, syphilis, and even scurvy (138). The lack of precision and overall general confusion regarding these skin diseases is nicely summarized by the London physician Thomas Spooner's comment in 1728 that, 'The Itch and Scabies are usually the forerunners of [leprosy], for the Itch, being neglected, turns to an universal Scabies, and that to the Leprosy as before

shewn, which is the worst of the cutaneous diseases, and accompanied with the highest degree of corruption and putrefaction.' (210)

14. Even today medical parlance is replete with arcane terms that lack specificity; for example, 'rheumatism'.

15. In his 1868 writing *On Diseases of the Skin*, von Hebra proclaimed:

> The name of 'scabies' is at the present day used to designate the numerous morbid appearances produced in the skin by the presence of the acari which dwell within it, and which, in obtaining food for themselves, and in propagating their species, give rise to a continual irritation of its component tissues. (27)

16. For example, von Hebra, wrote:

> Experience shows that in all persons who for a considerable time have been infested with acari (or, in other words, have had scabies) tubercles, or other appearances due to infiltration of the skin, arise on those parts of the body which are from any cause subjected to pressure or friction ... The first example I will give is that of men who sit for a long time together on hard stools or benches. In such persons, when they get the itch, there always appear on the buttocks, and exactly on those spots which correspond to the ischial tuberosities, either papules or tubercles, or pustules and crusts. On some of these tubercles, in the direction of their long axis, may be seen burrows; while others are simple elevations of the epidermis, and contain no parasite. Among the workmen who present these appearances, arising from the above-named cause, are, for instance, cobblers, tailors, and weavers; whereas carpenters, joiners, and bricklayers, all of whom work standing, and not sitting, remain free from anything of the kind, however severely they may be affected by the disease. A further confirmation of the view I am advocating may be found in the case of women who use straps or belts, whether as part of their ordinary wearing apparel, or to fasten things which they carry while at work. Whenever such belts or strings are allowed to exert pressure on the skin, the result is the formation, at the affected spots, of the tubercles above described, with or without burrows on their summits. Precisely similar effects, again, follow the irritation caused by using trusses or crutches, or by wearing garters, girdles, or, indeed, tight clothes of any kind whatever. (27)

17. In 1916, the centennial year of von Hebra's birth, the medical historian Victor Robinson wrote:

> This is the centennial year of Hebra's birth. A century is sufficient to swallow up most human beings. Millions were born in 1816—how many are remembered in 1916? But dermatologists—and who among us is not something of a dermatologist—can celebrate the centenary of a name that will not be wiped out by the flood of time: for dermatology knows no greater name than that of Ferdinand von Hebra. (135)

18. The mid-nineteenth-century American dermatologist James Clark White, who studied with von Hebra, expressed his progressive knowledge of scabies writing in Boston in 1864, 'The use of internal remedies belongs to the days when a belief in a dyscrasy prevailed, and nothing need be said about it' (84). Louis Duhring, professor of Dermatology at University of Pennsylvania, and perhaps the preeminent American dermatologist of the nineteenth century was also a pupil of von Hebra's, Today von Hebra's bust accompanies that of Sigmund Freud, and another famous dermatologist, Moriz Kaposi, at the office of the dean of the medical faculty at the University of Vienna. (133)

8

Therapy

Richard

Richard came to see me, itchy and scratched up. A man in his mid-80s, he recently had been treated for eczema with topical steroids and oral antibiotics, but was not getting better. A cursory examination revealed a frail-appearing man with plenty of scabs and a fair amount of bruising. More detailed inspection with the dermatoscope revealed what I suspected to be a burrow. A quick scraping and a trip to the microscope where I visualized a mite confirmed my suspicions.

'You have scabies, and I have just the medication to make you better', I dutifully informed him. Richard seemed a bit puzzled. 'I have what?' he asked. I repeated myself. 'Scabies? What's that, and how did I get it?' he inquired. Common questions which I sat down to answer. I confirmed he had no close contacts needing cotreatment, and then proceeded to discuss therapy. I told Richard to stop by the pharmacy and pick up a topical medication called permethrin, the current preferred treatment for scabies, which I instructed him to rub neck down all over his skin. 'Don't skip anywhere', I added. 'Be sure to get all the cracks and crevices—in between your fingers and toes, in your armpits and groin—all body folds; and be sure to thoroughly treat your penis and scrotum.'

Richard looked at me in silence for a few seconds, trying to process all of that mouthful, and then headed off to the pharmacy. I washed up and headed to see my next patient. Then back to my office for the obligatory electronic paperwork. Then to see the next case. Then to the next. More charting, then to the next. Perhaps 45 minutes transpired when my medical assistant knocked on the door, and I briefly excused myself from the room. 'Richard is back, and he has more questions', she told me. 'Sure thing', I replied, 'Please put him back in a room.' After finishing up with my patient, I popped in the adjacent exam room to see Richard and address his additional questions. He was holding a tube of permethrin. 'Yep, that's the right stuff', I exclaimed. Richard looked at me somewhat baffled, 'I don't think I can use this. I don't know how to use it.

I don't even know where to begin', he replied. 'Well, it's simple, you squirt some out on your hand and rub all around your neck, and then work your way down', I gestured. 'But I've never done it before. There are so many places that I cannot reach. I would much prefer if you do it', he beseeched.

Unusual request, I thought, but here we both are, so why not? Oral therapy for scabies now exists, but he had the topical antiscabies treatment in his hand. I suppose I could have delegated the task to someone else but why not engage in hands on healing? I stepped out while he disrobed, donning a cloth gown, and when I came back in I gloved up, removed his robe, and applied the permethrin into his every skin crack and crevice. It reminded me a bit of being rubbed down in a Turkish hammam, but I took it even further. Scrotum to the left, scrotum to the right, perineum, penile shaft, head of the penis. Viola! And when he came back in 4 weeks, Richard was cured.

Treatment

Since the days of the ancient Greek physician Galen, physicians approached The Itch as a disease requiring systemic or internal treatment. Topical treatments were frowned upon as they were thought to drive the malady back into the body preventing its full cure. Thus standard therapies would often include bloodletting, purges, or a variety of ingestible concoctions of dubious repute. Irrespective of the approach used, many early treatments for scabies likely carried some degree of toxicity. In some instances they could confer adverse effects far worse than The Itch itself. In the eighteenth century, the English physician Thomas Spooner described employing a quicksilver girdle, a mercury laden tight fitting garment, to cure The Itch, which led to a series of unintended consequences due to mercury poisoning.[1]

> A lusty matron (says Hildanus) about forty years old, fat, and of a moist constitution of body, when in the month of February, she had put on a quicksilver girdle for a small itch, and had worn it for three weeks day and night, she indeed was rid of her itch, but there followed a salivation, exulceration of the gums, and heaviness in the head, which was followed by a catarrh on the left side, and weakness of the same. (210)

When physician prescribed treatments proved unsuccessful, sufferers turned to a variety of alternate healers, or as specified by von Hebra, 'quacks and old women' (27). In cases where there was awareness of the mite proper, physically removing them one by one with a fine needle proved popular, especially amongst the poorer classes. Others employed various oral, topical, or combination therapies that were messy, potentially toxic, and often ineffective. The irony of it all, was that an effective treatment for scabies, sulphur, had been known since antiquity.

Sulphur and Other Early Treatments

The Roman author Celsus, in the first century AD, recommended a mixture of sulphur and pitch, a tarry distillate, for the cure of human and animal scabies. Around the same time, the Roman author Columella noted that, 'wild marjoram and sulphur, bruised together and boiled in lees of oil mixed with oil, water, and vinegar' was a remedy for animal scabies. Presumably the use of sulphur for treating The Itch far predates this description. Treatment with sulphur, however, was often highly disagreeable, being messy, potentially malodorous (depending on the exact form used), and damaging to clothing. In his treatise on the subject of scabies, Spooner mentions the use of brimstone (sulphur) taken internally and used externally as an ointment for treatment 'according to the vulgar method', but lamented:

> that it obliges those who take and use it, either to confine themselves during the whole course, or else to let every one they come near, know they are troubled with The Itch; for the smell of it is so very strong, as not to be overcome, or be concealed, from even those who only just pass by the persons who use it, much less from them they converse with, to whom it smells much more plain, strong, and filthy than to themselves. (210)

Perhaps this was one of the reasons that its therapeutic use was neglected and somewhat forgotten, only to be revisited in the eighteenth century.[2] In the nineteenth and early twentieth century, however, sulphur as the treatment for The Itch made a comeback, and eventually became regarded as the mainstay of therapy for scabies. Numerous variations and modifications to the sulphur treatment of scabies were proposed to make it more tolerable.

The main medical drawback of sulphur is that it is a skin irritant. When used topically, sulphur can cause a caustic chemical burn, a reaction known as an irritant contact dermatitis, as well as an itchy eruption mimicking scabies itself, known as an allergic contact dermatitis. When treating scabies, not infrequently the resulting sulphur irritation can be more debilitating than the original itch itself. Thus sulphur had to be used carefully, and while effective against scabies, was not an ideal treatment.

Sulphur-induced dermatitis was treated through use of soothing starch bathes and other mollifying topical applications, none of which would have been particularly effective. Mainly, time and avoidance of additional sulphur application would be the recipe for cure. Yet, patients and physicians alike often would mistake sulphur dermatitis for the scabietic itch itself, and thus retreat with additional rounds of sulphur, leading to a miserable endless cycle. Severe cases of sulphur irritancy could take months to resolve. Often physicians were callous to the detrimental effects of sulphur treatment, with the view that the ends justified the means. von Hebra, again, was quick to critique their methods, pointing out that:

> … veterinary surgeons have in this matter paid more respect to the skin and hair of their patients than medical men have to theirs. This, indeed, is not surprising, for the fleeces of sheep, and the skins of other animals, have a far higher market value than is possessed by the integument of a man who has The Itch! (27)

In its elemental state, sulphur is an inert and odourless compound. By various purification methods it can be rendered into different preparations (precipitated, sublimated, or washed), and combined with a vehicle to form a salve for medical treatment. One of the earliest and simplest formulations was that of Joseph Frank (1771–1842) who mixed equal parts sulphur into butter. Along similar lines, Sir John Pringle, an early proponent of military hygiene, treated scabietic soldiers with one part sulphur mixed in two parts lard. With time, more sophisticated preparations were fashioned, in an attempt to make the concoction less disagreeable. von Hebra notes that Bourguignon's formula of sulphur, potassium carbonate, gum tragacanth, glycerine, and oils of lavender, carnation, menthol, and cinnamon would 'probably be very useful in practice among the higher classes, on account of its agreeable smell'. However he noted that of the many various sulphur preparations hyped by physicians and druggists, all were similar in efficacy.[3]

One approach to minimizing sulphur irritancy was to restrict treatment only to the specific itchy areas of the body. At the Hôpital St. Louis in Paris, the eminent dermatologist Pierre Louis Alphee Cazenave[4] treated scabietics under his care with a sulphur salve rubbed merely into affected patients' wrists, hands, and feet. This limited application method required multiple rounds of treatment and was associated with a high failure rate. His successor,

Pierre-Antoine-Ernest Bazin, treated patients' entire integument, from head to toe, and was far more effective, requiring only two rounds of treatment for cure. Based on this experience, a variety of total body treatment rapid cure protocols were devised and tested. The technique of sulphur fumigation was attempted but abandoned because of lack of efficacy combined with severe sulphur dermatitis. A technique called the English method, proved more successful, and is described by von Hebra as follows:

> The patient was first put in a bath, and washed all over with soap, and he was then rubbed with a sulfur-ointment, and placed naked in bed between two blankets. Here he was kept for forty-eight hours, during which time the room maintained at a constant temperature of 77F, whatever the season of the year. The frictions were repeated every morning and evening, and he was made to drink warm fluids freely, so as to increase the cutaneous perspiration.

This method, while being effective, also led to severe sulphur dermatitis (14). In addition, the washing of bed and blankets, as well as the heating required, incurred considerable expense. Removal of the heating component led to what was termed the 'modified English method', which reduced the cost of the treatment but did not ameliorate the sulphur dermatitis. Further improvement was devised by Hardy, whose method of 'rapid treatment' von Hebra describes as follows:

> The patient, having been placed in a warm bath, is rubbed vigorously with black soap for half an hour; he remains in the bath for another hour, at the end of which time he is taken out of the water and has Helmerich's [sulphur] ointment rubbed forcibly into the whole surface of the body. This terminates the treatment, the patient, before being discharged, being merely told to take a few warm bathes.[5]

Ultimately, the goal was to find a highly effective treatment that was quick, easy, and of minimal expense. The method as devised by Vlemingkx came to be regarded as the most widely applicable. Even von Hebra adopted its use.

> The patient is first to be placed in a bath, in which he is rubbed all over vigorously for half an hour with pieces of coarse flannel and with potass soap, or even common washing soap. He is to be told beforehand that this part of the treatment is of great importance, since it exposes the burrows of the itch-mite, softens the epidermis, and enables it to be more easily penetrated by

the solution of sulfuret of calcium which will afterwards be applied. After the soap has been well rubbed in, the patient is left for another half-hour in the bath. During the third half-hour he is again rubbed all over, and no less forcibly than before, with pieces of flannel, which, however, are now dipped in the solution of sulfuret of calcium. The fourth half-hour (which completes the period of time devoted to the cure of the disease) is again passed in the bath. At its expiration, any particles of sulphur that may still adhere to the skin may be washed off with cold water, or by means of the douche. Clean linen should then, if possible, be given him to wear, and this terminates the course of treatment. In the Belgian army, Vlemingkx's method is carried out in such a way that a soldier sent to the hospital for scabies does not even have his name taken off the list of effectives.

While this method seems like nothing more than a vigorous rubdown with a sulphurized buf-puf, it had the important advantage of being highly effective and could be widely utilized in military settings. It soon became the official scabies treatment for the Belgian army, and was adopted by other militaries as well. Those having undergone the treatment, however, often looked worse after the fact because of the severe sulphur dermatitis it caused. According to von Hebra, 'in the eyes of a lay observer such a patient will not appear to have been cured'. With a treatment time of but 2 hours, troops were immediately sent back to their units without additional time afforded for recuperation. Needless to say, this method was not recommended for paying private clients nor for those 'who have red or fair hair, whose skin is delicate, and in whom (as is well known) irritation of the skin is more commonly followed by severe effects'.

Exactly how does sulphur work in treating scabies? Surprisingly, the exact mechanism still remains a mystery. Sulphur as compounded into salves is an inert compound. Mellanby showed that the scabies mite can survive for days in sulphur ointment on a glass slide (85). Erasmus Wilson in 1846 postulated that sulphur 'probably combines with hydrogen, and sulfuretted hydrogen gas is evolved, which acts as a deadly poison', killing the mite and its eggs. Friedman (14) proposed that sulphur might have antiscabietic properties through a multistep oxidative process culminating in the formation of a chemical called pentathionic acid. It is very likely that a component of the skin activates sulphur into its scabicidal form. Irrespective of its actual mechanism, sulphur treatment of scabies has shown great durability; only recently has it been supplanted by other newer treatments. Scabies and sulphur, through their long history will always be connected, not unlike syphilis and mercury. In fact, sulphur is still routinely employed where cost is the predominant consideration

(7), and remains the officially recommended treatment of choice during pregnancy and lactation (1).

Over the centuries, hundreds, perhaps thousands, of alternative treatments for scabies have been utilized. Initially, natural products have provided the inspiration and the raw materials for these numerous topical preparations. An early example of this comes from none other than Bonomo and Cestoni. In their landmark treatise of 1687, they recommended treating scabies with tobacco leaves. Numerous additional examples exist; of which only a few of the more notable will be described here. One of the most widely used has been Balsam of Peru, the sap of the tree *Myroxylon balsamum var. pereirae*. This tree grows in Central America and historically was collected by the Spanish and sent to Peru from where it was shipped to Europe, thereby acquiring its moniker. Specifically, one of its constituent components, benzyl benzoate, has been and continues to be successfully used to treat scabies (48). Mainly because of its low cost, it remains a popular scabicide in many developing nations to this day.

Another plant found to have antiscabietic properties was the derris root, originally used by natives of the Amazon as a natural insecticide. It is an effective scabicide when mixed with water and applied to the skin (87), or it can be further purified to its active ingredient rotenone. Other natural products used to treat scabies which have more recently attracted much interest include tea tree oil from the Australian native plant *Melaleuca alternifolia* (43). And any such list of course must include the chrysanthemum flower, and its related active ingredients the pyrethrins. From pyrethrins, chemists have derived permethrin, the cornerstone of modern day topical scabies treatment in the United States and much of the industrialized world.

Lindane

After sulphur, the next advances in the topical treatment of scabies came from the petrochemical industry. Early on, pure petroleum had been advocated as an alternative to sulphur treatments for scabies, by Montgomery and Culver, who found it 'a quick and effective scabicide ... [with] ... the disadvantage that ... all the patients have to wear petroleum-soaked gloves, shorts, drawers and socks for several days, during which time, of course, they constitute dangerous fire hazards' (14). A further refinement came in the form of hexachlorocyclohexane, which was studied by Thomas in the early 1940s for its insecticidal properties. It was found that one of the geometrical configurations of this compound, the gamma isomer, was an effective veterinary insecticide.

Topical 1% gamma-hexachlorocyclohexane was further investigated and de-termined to have potent activity against the scabies mite. Even more important was that it caused minimal to no skin irritancy, a distinct improvement over the use of sulphur (86, 197). The gamma isomer was thus termed 'gammexane' (and later 'lindane'), and developed for commercial use. Its primary mech-anism of action is that it causes neurotoxicity, leading scabies mites to seize and die. Lindane rapidly gained acceptance and at the height of its use, over one million prescriptions were dispensed per year (45).

Unfortunately, under various circumstances, lindane was found to cause neurotoxicity in humans as well. The first inkling of this occurred in 1951 when 79 persons in the Greek town of Carpenissi fell ill after exposure to an insecticidal powder that they had sprinkled on the grounds and walls of their houses. The powder used was 40% hexachlorocyclohexane, containing a com-bination of the alpha, gamma, and delta isomers. Those affected developed diz-ziness, torpor, headache, and body aches, followed by diarrhoea, mouth sores, and neurological symptoms. Six deaths ensued (32). The drug was found to be highly fat soluble preferentially accumulating in the lipid-rich white matter of the brain. From 1960 to 1977, 26 cases of toxicity were reported from the use of topical 1% lindane used to treat scabies (45). Considering that an estimated 24 million applications were utilized during this time period, this is a very small number. However, these included instances of seizure and death, even after a single application. Infants and young children were found to be particularly susceptible (193). Based on a growing appreciation of its potential for toxicity, a lengthy and somewhat impractical set of guidelines for safe use of lindane was suggested, including (i) avoidance of use after a hot bath which might promote internal absorption; (ii) avoidance of repeat application in a short time span; (iii) avoidance in conjunction with oils or oil based preparations; (iv) avoid-ance in children where thumb sucking or licking would be likely; (v) extreme caution in excoriated skin or skin with an epidermal barrier defect; (vi) contra-indication to use in neonates and children or adults with a history of seizure disorders; (vii) avoidance in conjunction with occlusive diapers, shower caps, or tight clothes; (viii) avoidance of reapplication within 6 hours; (ix) avoidance of breast feeding within 24 hours of use; and (x) prohibition on pharmacists dispensing more than 2 fluid ounces of medication at a time.

The risk of extremely rare but serious injury as a result of topical treatment for scabies was not something that most were willing to stomach. The list of precautionary steps suggested rendered the safe use of lindane prohibitively burdensome and impractical to all but the most detail-oriented. With the advent of other agents having a more favourable safety profile, in particular the chrysanthemum derivative permethrin, in 1995, the US Food and Drug Administration classified lindane as 'second-line' therapy for scabies. Because of its questionable impact on children, as well as concerns regarding lindane pollution of the water supply, this pesticide was banned outright by the state of California in 2002. Other countries have followed suit, though the medication is still available for use in parts of the United States, albeit with a black box warning. The Environmental Protection Agency and the World Health Organization both consider lindane to have 'moderate' acute toxicity.

Permethrin

The product that would eventually supersede lindane use in the United States was permethrin, a chemically modified pyrethrin, one of the naturally occurring insecticides found in the chrysanthemum flower. Like lindane, permethrin is a highly effective scabicide with minimal risk for causing skin irritation, and it has an improved safety profile. It remains one of the most effective drugs to treat scabies, even today, with its main drawback being its cost.

Dried chrysanthemum flowers had long been known to carry insecticidal properties, and likely were used for such purposes by the Chinese as far back as the first century AD (53), around the same time that the Romans were using sulphur. Chrysanthemum flowers were used similarly in Persia, and introduced to Europe by Armenian traders around 200 years ago as 'Persian dust' (44, 53). Chrysanthemum (*Chrysanthemum cinerariaefolium*) flowers from Dalmatia (modern day Croatia), were found to have highly active insecticidal properties, and by the mid-nineteenth century were being grown and exported in large numbers. By the 1860s, bales of dried chrysanthemum flowers were imported into the United States and sold as 'Dalmatian insect powder'. Over the ensuing decades, these products attained widespread use, with a total of 3 million pounds being consumed by the United States in 1919.

Around this time it was realized that by soaking chrysanthemum flowers with kerosene one could extract out and concentrate the insecticidal activity. Further research performed by the chemists Staudinger and Ruzicka identified two primary active agents in the flower—pyrethrin I and II (50). More specifically, it was found that *Chrysanthemum cinerariaefolium* contained six active pyrethrin components formed by the combination of chrysanthemic acid (pyrethrin I fraction) and pyrethric acid (pyrethrin II fraction) with three alcohols—pyrethrolone, cinerolone, and jasmolone. The chemist Gnadiger discovered a method for quantifying the amount of pyrethrin in the dried flowers or their extracts, and it was determined that *Chrysanthemum cinerariaefolium* grown in Kenya, where a local cultivation industry was encouraged, produced flowers with the highest pyrethrin concentration. Initial use of pyrethrin was most often geared to combating mosquitoes, fleas, or body lice as well as agricultural pests. Because of its relative instability to light and heat, frequent reapplication was required to maintain its insecticidal effects.

World War I interrupted ready access to the Dalmatian market, and other sources for chrysanthemum flowers were needed. Initially the Japanese market proved able to support the demand. Within 2 decades the Japanese were producing 28 million pounds of chrysanthemum (50). The onset of World War II yet again interrupted the global chrysanthemum trade. Not only did the main supply come from Japan, an Axis power, but increasingly military applications for this product were recognized, particularly in protecting troops from malaria and other insect-borne diseases. The US government commandeered all available supplies for military use (44), and alternate suppliers under Allied control were sought. By this point, African production had ramped up considerably with Kenya, Tanzania, and the Belgian Congo now providing the majority of Allied demand.

In 1941, the entomologists Lyle Goodhue and William Sullivan successfully determined a method to dispense pyrethrins with liquified gas from a one pound portable refillable cylinder, which became colloquially known as the 'bug bomb'. Chlorofluorocarbons were used as the gaseous agent predominantly, as they were inert and originally thought to be nontoxic and harmless (only much later would their detrimental effect on the ozone be discovered). The birth of the modern spray allowed US soldiers to 'debug' their environment and protect themselves from malarial mosquitoes and other disease carrying insects. It was estimated that at least 40 million of these canisters were utilized in World War II. This was one of the earliest applications of aerosol technology, for which they received a patent in 1943 (44). Only after World War II did the potential of pyrethrin in treating scabies become recognized.

Beginning in the mid-1950s, importation shifted from chrysanthemum flowers in bulk to strictly their resinous extracts. These extracts contained high levels of pyrethrins (30%), leading to considerable savings on shipping costs. In the meantime, scientific advances allowed for the complete chemical characterization of the various pyrethrins, such that resources could be allocated to developing a synthetic stable version of these compounds for mass commercial use. The ultimate goal was to find an effective and safe synthetic product which would render unnecessary any reliance on the agriculture and transportation industries. After several attempts, in 1973, a synthetic pyrethroid was developed with a good toxicity profile, increased potency, and good stability in the presence of light. This product was termed 'permethrin' (176). Permethrin had the distinct advantage over pyrethrin in that it maintains activity for up to 2 weeks in direct sunlight. Initially clinical investigations of permethrin were undertaken in Egypt to combat body lice, which had locally acquired considerable resistance against the pesticide DDT (177). In these early studies, permethrin was shown to be a safe and effective insecticide. Permethrin was also found to be effective at treating both human and rat fleas. Studies were subsequently performed showing 1% permethrin to be safe and effective against head lice. Comparatively it was found to be more effective than over-the-counter products containing pyrethrin extract (many of which are still available on the market today) (178). Eventually 1% permethrin would gain US Food and Drug Administration approval for the treatment of head lice and be sold under the trade name NIX in the United States, and Lyclear in other countries. Permethrin was also shown to be efficacious for the treatment of crabs (pubic lice). In addition to its direct use to treat skin or hair infested parasites, permethrin was found to have utility in the treatment of netting, tents, curtains, screens, and clothing (including military uniforms) to kill and deter the presence of biting insects which are responsible for vector-borne illness, such as malaria. As of 1989, synthetic permethrin accounted for 25% of the world insecticide market.

Given its efficacy on lice, the use of permethrin on other parasites was further explored. Studies on scabies were performed in 1983 on populations in Panama, where scabies had been endemic for over a decade. In this population, for reasons not entirely clear, a high rate of lindane resistance was noted. Children were particularly impacted with over two-thirds being afflicted with scabies; many of these children also suffered from a variety of potentially more serious bacterial infections because of the chronic itching and scratching brought on by scabies. Initial studies found a single application of 5% permethrin to be highly effective in this population, curing more than 90% of all scabies cases after 4 weeks. In contrast, only 65% of lindane treated patients were cured at 4 weeks. Those who failed lindane treatment were switched to the permethrin treatment arm of the study and were all subsequently cured (179, 180, 44). The use of permethrin was without irritation, allergic reaction, or other side-effects, and was in general well-accepted, being cosmetically elegant and odourless, without staining clothing or other garments.

A larger multicentre clinical trial performed at various centres in the United States and Mexico of over 460 subjects was published in 1990, showing permethrin 5% cream to be equally or slightly more effective than lindane 1% in the treatment of scabies. Around this time 5% permethrin garnered official FDA approval for treatment of scabies. Given concerns about the rare albeit serious risks of neurotoxicity with lindane use (especially in children), permethrin, with its excellent safety profile, quickly vaulted itself to the topical drug of choice against scabies in the United States. Side-effects of 5% permethrin were transient and mild—consisting primarily of stinging or burning upon application. Internal absorption and accumulation in the body tissues was determined to be negligible, attributable to the fact that permethrin is almost entirely detoxified by enzymes present in the skin. After topical administration, permethrin could not be measured in the blood at a detectable level (44). Inactive metabolites were found to be excreted in the urine at a faster rate than absorbed into the bloodstream. Overall permethrin was found to have all the properties of an excellent scabicidal drug—except for its cost, which is considerably more than almost all other alternative treatments. This has unfortunately limited its use in much of the world; however, permethrin continues to be the treatment of choice for scabies in the United States to this day—so much so that many a modern day dermatologist has used permethrin, and only permethrin, to treat scabies and has utterly no experience using sulphur, benzyl benzoate, or lindane.

Permethrin and pyrethrins, like lindane, work by causing damage to the arthropod nervous system. Specifically they bind to invertebrate (but not vertebrate) ion channels, leading them to undergo repetitive discharges which lead to eventual paralysis and death (26). Permethrin thus acts as a selective neurotoxin. However, because of its great success as a drug and accompanying widespread use, a variety of arthropods have over time developed permethrin-resistance. And while permethrin resistant human scabies has not been formally documented, permethrin has been noted to take significantly longer to work in mite populations that have been subjected to extensive permethrin exposure (208). It is thus only a matter of time before the phenomenon of permethrin-resistance is observed in scabies.[6]

Ivermectin

Heretofore the discussion of scabies therapies has all revolved around topical treatments. Several millennia of experimentation with oral treatments, including orally ingested sulphur, had previously come to naught. The pioneers of scabies recognized this, and explicitly warned their disciples to avoid internal treatments and stick to external therapy. Bonomo and Cestoni admonished to avoid the 'rather fruitless results of internal treatment', while von Hebra lamented those patients 'tormented by a long course of internal medicines'. For The Itch, which had mysteriously afflicted so many, topical and topical treatment alone had been the route to cure. Until now. Pioneers such as von Hebra and the like, as well as more recent pupils of scabies such as Friedman, would surely sit up and take note that an effective oral treatment for scabies now exists. It goes by the name ivermectin.

Ivermectin did not start out its life as a drug to treat scabies; rather it was born of an attempt to discover novel veterinary drugs. The pharmaceutical giant Merck long had a division working on developing medications to treat intestinal parasites (such as tapeworm or hookworm), which affect humans, pets, and domestic animals alike. In the 1970s, to expand their drug-discovery efforts, Merck teamed up with the Kitasato Institute in Tokyo, Japan, which had developed and maintained a large stock of many thousand microbial cultures derived from soil samples obtained in Japan (196). Together they undertook an ambitious screening programme of these microbial cultures with the goal of isolating new compounds with veterinary potential.

To determine if any of these soil-derived cultures held promise, scientists at Merck added them to growth medium for 3 days, and the resultant broth was fed to worm-infested mice. Mice faeces were subsequently examined for the presence of worm eggs, and mice were sacrificed, and their intestines were microscopically examined for the presence of worms. Of all the Kitasato cultures studied, Merck investigators found one which appeared to have a protective effect. Infested mice that were fed this culture were found to be worm-free. Further purification revealed that this culture contained an unusual bacterium of the Actinomycete family called *Streptomyces avermitilis*. It was derived from a soil sample taken from a golf course near the Japanese city of Ito (63). Sophisticated chemical techniques, including thin-layer chromatography, led to the isolation of a group of compounds containing the antiparasitic property, and these were termed 'avermectins'. At the core of this word is the Latin 'vermes', meaning 'worm'. The hydrogenation product of one of these avermectins was found to have further advantageous properties, and this hydrogenated avermectin, 'hyvermectin', with a small nomenclature modification, became ivermectin, as we know today know it (61).

As hoped for, the avermectins, and ivermectin in particular, wound up having great utility as veterinary drugs. Ivermectin was noted to be effective against a variety of intestinal parasites in many different species of animals tested, including horses, sheep, goats, dogs, swine, and cattle. A topical formulation was found to be effective in treating rabbits whose ears were heavily infested with mites. Ivermectin proved itself to be effective, safe, and versatile, having not just antihelminthic activity (activity against intestinal worms) but also antiarthropod activity. Additional testing found it to be an effective internal medication against cattle scabies (*Sarcoptes scabiei var. bovis*) (211). With demonstration of efficacy in animals, it would only be a matter of time before a link to human scabies was made.

Before that would happen, however, ivermectin made a huge splash in a completely different arena. For centuries, subsistence farmers in certain areas of tropical Africa had suffered from a disease consisting of itchy skin lesions which over time evolved to thickened swollen areas of skin often with a loss of pigment—described as 'elephant skin' or 'leopard skin'. This condition, onchocerciasis, is due to a parasitic worm, *Onchocerca volvulus*. Larvae of the worm are transmitted by the bite of the blackfly *Simulium damnosum*, which breeds around fast flowing streams found predominantly in equatorial Africa. When a human is infected, larvae are deposited in the skin, mammary tissue, and lymph nodes, where they develop into adult worms and mate. The worms subsequently release additional larvae, or microfilaria, into the body and bloodstream, upon which they can travel to and lodge in other organs causing tissue inflammation. Such accumulations of microfilaria can lead to the formation of additional skin and subcutaneous nodules of all sizes called onchocercoma. In addition to involving the skin, over time, microfilaria accumulate in the eye, leading to progressive visual loss and eventual blindness. This disease has thus been called river blindness, and until recently, was one of the leading causes of acquired blindness worldwide. In some villages, it is estimated that 30%–50% of the population has been blinded (209). This severe disability has led to general impoverishment in these areas. Moreover, affected communities have been forced to abandon the richer fertile river valleys where the blackfly resides. Prior public health attempts at controlling it were mainly limited to spraying against the blackfly with DDT or other synthetic insecticides.

In its early days of development, ivermectin was found to be active against the larval (microfilarial) stages of dog heartworm but had no activity against the adult (macrofilarial) forms. This had several implications: (i) ivermectin could disrupt the heartworm lifecycle but not fully cure the disease and (ii) ivermectin turned out to possess an element of safety that other antiparasitics didn't. In controlling the disease, ivermectin left alone the adult forms and thus did not cause the massive inflammation that killing them could bring about. Moreover ivermectin did not cause the embolization, or lodging of adult worm fragments in the dog lung, which under certain circumstances could also be deadly. In short, ivermectin's microfilaricidal properties prevented it from being curative but enabled it to interrupt the parasitic lifecycle without causing massive end organ damage. For this reason, as well as the fact that it required continued treatment for its long-term efficacy, ivermectin was seen as a potential commercial boon, in particular as a heartworm medication.

In the course of ivermectin testing against gastrointestinal nematodes in horses, skin snippings were examined, almost as an afterthought, and ivermectin was found to be effective in killing the microfilaria of incidentally co-infected *Onchocerca cervicalis*, an esoteric horse parasite (211). This observation was extended to Onchocerca in cattle. Thus testing ivermectin against human onchocerciasis was logical. Clinical trials were embarked upon in 1981, and soon demonstrated that ivermectin also possessed selective microfilarial activity in the treatment of *Onchocerca volvulus* in humans. Similar to its action in dog heartworm, by lacking macrofilarial activity in humans, ivermectin could be employed without causing widespread tissue-destructive inflammation. Ultimately this meant that ivermectin could be used to disrupt the lifecycle of human onchocerciasis, while maintaining a relatively mild side-effect profile.

And in the treatment of human onchocerciasis alone, ivermectin has proven to be a wonder drug. Through widespread adoption and public health programmes, it has made a profound impact on treating and controlling river blindness worldwide. Owing to its success, in 1987 Merck pledged an open donation of ivermectin ('for as long as it might be needed') to the World Health Organization eradication programme, with the goal of eventual onchocerciasis elimination. It has been estimated that over 400 million people have been treated with ivermectin in Africa alone, likely saving millions from a life of blindness (26). Because it does not kill macrofilaria, maintenance ivermectin needs to be readministered to affected populations roughly every 6 months. This must be done for the lifespan of the adult worms, roughly 15–17 years, to prevent them from releasing microfilaria as the previously administered drug wears off. In spite of this limitation, ivermectin has been one of the most successful global public health programmes ever instituted (209). Moreover, ivermectin is active against a number of other medically important roundworms which infect humans, such as elephantiasis (lymphatic filariasis). For the development of this novel and important therapy, the investigators responsible for the discovery of ivermectin were awarded a share of the Nobel Prize in Physiology or Medicine in 2015.

While ivermectin proved to be remarkably successful in treating river blindness, it was also noted to have antiarthropod activity. Initially it was employed in cattle to treat a variety of ectoparasites including grubs, screwworms, lice, mites, and in some cases, ticks (61). In 1992 a random-ized blinded trial was performed in French Polynesia to assess the efficacy of oral ivermectin in treating human scabies comparing it with topical benzyl benzoate. It was found to be at least as effective a treatment. Moreover iver-mectin had the advantage of being administered as an oral formulation which certain individuals were more likely to use over topical treatment in the local hot and humid tropical conditions (75). Additional studies showed that ivermectin at a dose of 200 micrograms/kilogram was effective in curing many patients of scabies after a single dose, including some who some who were HIV+ (55).

Ivermectin was soon compared to permethrin in a head-on study. Surprisingly, it was found to be less effective. When taken as a single dose or application, ivermectin was shown to cure only 70%–90% of patients, whereas permethrin cured 95%–98% (35, 90). Further studies have validated the con-clusion that permethrin has a higher cure rate than ivermectin in the treatment of scabies (81). When a second dose of ivermectin is given, however, efficacy rates start to be become quite comparable (35, 98, 106).

Why permethrin is superior to ivermectin in the treatment of scabies is not clear. In the treatment of head lice, ivermectin is known to kill adult forms but harbours no activity against their eggs or nits (94, 97). Possibly a similar phenomenon exists in the case of scabies, specifically that ivermectin is not ef-fective on immature (nymphal/larval) stages in the lifecycle. It is possible that ivermectin in unable to penetrate through the shell of unhatched scabies eggs (35). A second dose of ivermectin at a 2-week interval brings its cure rate to 95%, near parity with that of permethrin (98). This second dose would poten-tially kill off previously immature mites which had subsequently moulted into full adults, before they could mate and extend the lifecycle.

Though ivermectin has a slightly lower cure rate in scabies compared to per-methrin, there are potential advantages to its use. For starters, it makes sense to use ivermectin in the case of permethrin failures, for whatever the reason. Ivermectin is additionally appealing for use in patients for whom widespread body application of permethrin poses difficulty or logistical challenges. This is particularly true when used in institutional settings, such as hospitals, nursing homes, or prisons. It also applies to patients with limited mobility or who for other medical reasons are not confidently able to treat their entire skin sur-face.[7] In addition, ivermectin is useful for treating cases of scabies that have a heavy mite burden, such as Norwegian scabies, which can be difficult to cure irrespective of treatment modality, and may benefit from multiple rounds of cotreatment with permethrin (Figure 8.1a & b).

(a)

(b)

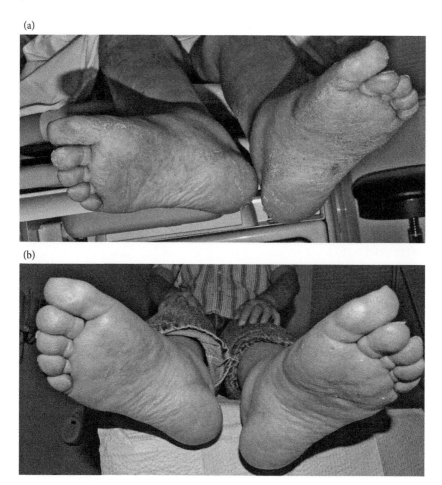

Figure 8.1a & b Crusted scabies before and after treatment with oral ivermectin.

When taking into account public health initiatives involving the mass treatment of endemic scabies, the tables are flipped, however, and ivermectin turns out to be more effective than permethrin. Particularly in developing tropical communities, a high percentage of the population can be affected by scabies at baseline. In such areas heavily impacted by scabies, due to the convenience of oral dosing, ivermectin is the superior antiscabietic drug. While mass permethrin administration reduced scabies infestation by two-thirds, mass ivermectin administration (provided as a single dose for most participants with a second dose for scabies infected individuals) virtually eradicated scabies, clearing more than 95% of cases, and dramatically reduced the secondary skin infections associated with scabies (89, 113).

How does ivermectin work? Similar to permethrin, ivermectin affects the ability of nerve cells to fire properly by binding to and disrupting ion channels.[8] And similar to permethrin, it has an excellent safety profile. This has been confirmed from a wealth of data from its extensive use in Africa, with the most common side-effect being itching (68). Oral ivermectin is currently not recommended for use in children younger than 5 years of age, though given its extensive use and excellent safety profile, it has been suggested that it is permissible to use in children weighing more than 15 kilograms. Recent data suggest that oral ivermectin is safe in infants and children weighing less than 15 kilograms as well (153). Ivermectin is not recommended for use in pregnancy, though inadvertent administration to over 400 pregnant women in their first trimester in an onchocerciasis control programme did not lead to an increase in birth defects (67).

Ivermectin resistance has been detected in nematodes but to date has not yet been noted in mites, or other arthropods in nature (96). And like with permethrin, there is reason to believe that ivermectin resistant scabies mites could one day become a clinical reality. Analysis of mites from patients with recurrent and severe Norwegian scabies reveals the drug works less well after multiple rounds of treatment. A drastic increase is noted in the time required for ivermectin to be scabicidal (40). Lest we get overly complacent, there is a continued need for research and development of antiscabietic drugs.

Treatment Failure

Failure to cure scabies is a frustrating experience for patient and physician alike. When patients fail to improve after treatment, a reassessment of the case is imperative. One must first ask, is this truly a case of scabies? This is particularly germane when microscopic confirmation is lacking, and clear-cut burrows have not been established. Scabies can be tricky to diagnose, particularly in atypical cases. Mellanby's finding that most individuals harbour six or less mites makes the task even more daunting. Moreover, there are plenty of other itchy skin conditions out there. In some cases, if such a patient is not getting better, one very real possibility is that they have something other than scabies (Table 8.1).

Consensus Criteria have been proposed to help standardize the diagnosis of scabies, and involve classifying the certainty that any given case is scabies. The International Alliance for the Control of Scabies has put forth three main

Table 8.1 Differential Diagnosis of Scabies

Differential Diagnoses for Typical Lesions of Common Scabies	Differential Diagnoses for Specific Scabies Signs and Variant Presentations
Arthropod bites	Burrows
Atopic dermatitis	Cutaneous larva migrans
Avian mites	Larva currens
Contact dermatitis, irritant or allergic	Infantile scabies
Delusionary parasitosis	Infantile acropustulosis
Dermatitis herpetiformis	Urticaria pigmentosa
Dyshidrotic eczema (pompholyx)	Bullous scabies
Erythroderma (exfoliative eczema)	Bullous arthropod bites
Fiberglass dermatitis	Bullous drug eruptions
Folliculitis	Bullous impetigo
Impetigo	Bullous pemphigoid
Langerhans cell histiocytosis	Incontinentia pigmenti
Lice: body and pubic	(inflammatory stage)
Lichen planus	Pemphigus vulgaris
Nummular (discoid) eczema	Crusted scabies
Molluscum contagiosum	Atopic dermatitis
Mycosis fungoides	Contact dermatitis
Onchocerciasis (acute and chronic	Darier disease
papular onchodermatitis)	Erythrodermic mycosis fungoides or
Papular urticaria	Sézary syndrome
Pityriasis rosea	Palmoplantar keratoderma
Prurigo nodularis	Pityriasis rubra pilaris
Secondary syphilis	Psoriasis
Tinea (corporis, manuum, or pedis)	Seborrhoeic dermatitis
Transient acantholytic dermatosis	
Verrucas (warts)	
Varicella zoster (chickenpox, shingles)	
Viral exanthems	

Reproduced under the STM agreement from Engelman, D. et al. (2020) The 2020 International Alliance for the Control of Scabies Consensus Criteria for the Diagnosis of Scabies. British Journal of Dermatology. 183: 808–820. https://doi.org/10.1111/bjd.18943.

categories which are useful in this regard: confirmed scabies, clinical scabies, and suspected scabies (92, 156) (Box 8.1).

Confirmed scabies can be defined as cases in which the scabies mite, its eggs, or faeces have been definitively detected. This can be accomplished using a desktop microscope, another high-powered imaging device, or a dermatoscope (a hand-held surface microscope). In short, rendering a diagnosis of confirmed scabies requires equipment and expertise. When confirmed cases of scabies do not respond to treatment, the inclination is often to cast blame on the medication used. However, drug resistance, while not impossible, is unlikely to be the root cause. The specifics of how the treatment was administered need to be

---

Box 8.1 The 2020 International Alliance for the Control of Scabies Criteria for the Diagnosis of Scabies. These criteria are for classical scabies and are not meant to be used for cases of crusted (Norwegian) scabies. B and C are useful when a microscope, dermatoscope, or other sophisticated equipment is not available for clinical use

---

A. Confirmed scabies

   At least one of:

   A1: Mites, eggs, or faeces on light microscopy of skin samples

   A2: Mites, eggs, or faeces visualized on an individual using a high-powered imaging device

   A3: Mite visualized on an individual using dermoscopy

B. Clinical scabies

   At least one of:

   B1: Scabies burrows

   B2: Typical lesions affecting male genitalia

   B3: Typical lesions in a typical distribution and two history features

C. Suspected scabies

   One of:

   C1: Typical lesions in a typical distribution and one history feature

   C2: Atypical lesions or atypical distribution and two history features

History features

   H1: Itch

   H2: Positive contact history

Reproduced under the STM agreement from Engelman, D. et al. (2020) The 2020 International Alliance for the Control of Scabies Consensus Criteria for the Diagnosis of Scabies. British Journal of Dermatology. 183: 808–820. https://doi.org/10.1111/bjd.18943.

Diagnosis can be made at one of the three levels (A, B, or C). A diagnosis of clinical or suspected scabies should only be made if other differential diagnoses are considered less likely than scabies.

---

analysed in greater detail, as incomplete use of the medication or failure to co-treat close contacts is often responsible.

Clinical scabies, on the other hand, are cases that lack a smoking gun, but have all the otherwise characteristic features. Cases lacking definitive confirmation, but having the classic signs of either burrows, or red bumps on the penis or scrotum (diagnostic for scabies unless proven otherwise) are considered clinically scabies. After this, what is and isn't considered clinical scabies depends on specifically defined criteria. A patient can be considered to have clinical scabies if they have 'typical lesions in a typical distribution' and have the two major clinical features of scabies: (i) they must be itchy and (ii) they must have close contact with someone else who has a similar itchy presentation. When these patients fail to improve with therapy, they also should be re-evaluated with an additional push to confirming the diagnosis. If possible, repeated skin examination with a dermatoscope and multiple additional skin scrapings are warranted to search for evidence of the mite.

Lastly, suspected scabies is a category that can be applied to cases that aren't better explained by another disease process, and that have some features of scabies. This enables the clinician to maintain an index of suspicion in the absence of key defining features. Suspected scabies is defined as 'typical lesions in a typical distribution' with only one major clinical feature (itch or close contacts having a similar presentation), or 'atypical lesions in an atypical distribution' with both major clinical features.[9] When untreated, suspected scabies cases can eventually turn into clinical or confirmed scabies, at which point they may develop more classical features. Or such cases can clear with appropriate scabies therapy, and then a more resolute diagnosis is made, but only in retrospect. When cases of suspected scabies fail to clear, the same questions must be asked regarding whether close contacts were treated and whether scabies therapy was used properly. Retreatment, switching, or even combining therapeutic agents can be worth trying; however, one must be willing to accept the possibility that these cases are not scabies after all. Re-evaluation with additional measures, including skin biopsy, are often required for further characterization.

When a patient with confirmed scabies is treated with topical medication and fails to improve, it is worth examining in more detail exactly how the topical medication was used. In adults, for topical medication to be fully effective, it must be applied neck down and rubbed into the entire skin surface.[10] Any measure that interrupts or interferes with medication getting to high mite-burden areas, the fingers and wrists in particular, can lead to treatment failure. Examples of such behaviour include excessive handwashing in adults, or skin licking in young children. Prescribing insufficient quantity of medication is another prime reason that the skin may be not wind up being fully treated. Additionally attention should be paid to fingernails (and toenails), which should be trimmed short, and medication should be applied under the free edge of the nails—failure to do has been reported to lead to lack of treatment efficacy (46, 192). And when it is said that the entire skin surface needs to be treated, this includes all areas irrespective of whether they are itchy or not. Here, not uncommonly, confusion can occur, as patients have been known even with explicit instructions to only treat itchy or rashed areas. As Cazenave discovered in Paris nearly 2 centuries ago in the course of his sulphur investigations, partial application of topical treatment leads to a poor cure rate. Thus ideally patients should be provided with explicit written instructions in a language they understand detailing the proper use of topical treatments: in adults topical medicine should be applied everywhere neck down to the entire integument, including genitalia, whether lesions are present or not. The English physician and entomologist John O'Donel Alexander, author of an entire volume entitled *Arthropods and the Human Skin* (60), provides specific guidance on this point, in his extremely thorough chapter on scabies:

> Personal experience over more than 40 years has shown that it is not enough to tell the patient to apply the medicament to the whole body from the chin to the toes. Even this simple instruction is frequently misinterpreted, the principal mistake being to think that it applies only to lesions. It has therefore been the present writer's practice to instruct patients as follows: Apply the remedy to the whole body below the collar line. Start with the fingers, the spaces between the fingers, the hands and the wrists and rub in the medicament thoroughly. Then do the same to the forearms, the upper arms, the armpits, axillary folds, shoulders and back and front of the trunk. Women should pay particular attention to the breasts and nipple areas and men and boys to the external genitalia. The buttocks, thighs, lower legs, soles of the feet and the toes should finally be treated. All these areas should be treated whether there are any spots to be seen or not so that no part of the body mentioned is left untreated.

When topical medication is used in this fashion in a true case of scabies, it is almost always successful. This is true regardless of whether it is ovicidal or not. Hypothetically a second application may be required 1 week after the first. This is particularly important in cases of scabies with a high mite burden, as the second application will kill any newly hatched mites before they have a chance to mate and re-establish the scabies lifecycle. In cases of Norwegian scabies, where mites are often encrusted in thick scale, additional topical agents that assist in dissolving this scale (by breaking down keratin) may be required. Multiple rounds of permethrin may in fact be needed in such cases.

The next most common reason for failure to cure when using medication properly is failure to treat close contacts or others who might harbour the scabies mite. When close contacts such as a sexual partner or child are asymptomatic, it can be easy, or sometimes just convenient, to overlook the fact that they require concurrent treatment. Yet it is well-established that close contacts who are not treated can eventually spread scabies back to the original person they caught it from. Depending on how long the period of sensitization takes, up to a 2-month delay is possible between catching scabies and developing itch. Close contacts who have no rash or are not itchy very possibly constitute cases of scabies-in-progress.

To treat close contacts, it is imperative that physicians actively inquire about the patient's social and living circumstances. It is not uncommon for physicians to fail to do so, narrowly viewing their obligation as being to their patient alone. One must remember that scabies is not so much a disease of the individual but rather a disease of the individual and his or her immediate environment or community. Physicians, therefore, must actively recommend that close contacts be treated, and must prescribe appropriate quantities of medications for these individuals, even if they have not seen them personally. These are nontrivial barriers to change in standard medical practice that need to be addressed. At times asymptomatic close contacts may balk at the idea of treatment and need to be actively persuaded. To these individuals treatment can come across as unnecessary, inconvenient, impractical, costly, or downright embarrassing. The stigma of having scabies, or being treated for it, is understandable and certainly not new. The English physician Thomas Spooner writing nearly 3 centuries ago detailed the embarrassment associated with The Itch: 'To these reasons, why person miss of being entirely cured, we may add that those afflicted with The Itch etc. are for the most part ashamed to own it' (210).

Even in well-documented cases where all the requisite steps in treatment have been followed to the letter, it is not uncommon for patients to remain itchy for a surprisingly long time. In such cases, the natural worry is that one is dealing with a widely resistant superbug. The phenomenon of itching that continues after treatment has been properly applied, also known as postscabies pruritus, is not uncommon. Even though the mites in the skin have been killed, it takes time for the skin to turn over and slough off. During this time, the immune system does not discriminate between living and dead scabies. And even after complete slough has occurred, immunological memory can lead to persistent itch, (though 24 hours after effective therapy, the treated patient is no longer contagious (189)). In almost all persons this immune hypersensitivity will wane, though in some it can take months. Various individuals who are already predisposed to a vigorous itch-scratch cycle, such as those who suffer from eczema, can be particularly prone to postscabietic pruritus (188). A variety of anti-itch (and even immune-suppressing) regimens can be helpful in getting these individuals 'over the hump'. It is not unheard of for the itch of scabies to last 3 months after full cure, a distressing and apprehensive time period.

And lastly, the itch of scabies can occasionally live on as a sort of psychological trauma. There is an unfortunate subset of individuals who are so distressed by their experience with scabies, they live in a prolonged state of dread that they continue to harbour this infestation. Either because of prolonged hypersensitivity or other neurological mechanisms, their body is tricked into thinking they are continually infested. Such patients often go to extreme and irrational measures to rid themselves of The Itch—from dispensing of all their possessions, to treating themselves with caustic chemicals. Often for them scabies morphs into what can best be described as acarophobia. When such patients have poor insight, cannot be soothed, and develop delusional ideas, functional impairment occurs. Needless to say, this represents a most difficult problem.

Notes

1. Sir John Pringle in his 1753 military treatise *Observation on the Diseases of the Army in Camp and Garrison* noted that mercury was an ineffective treatment for scabies, pointing out that he had treated several syphilitics with internally ingested mercury to the point of 'complete salivation' without curing them of their concurrent itch (77).

   Today we recognize and regard mercury primarily as a historical treatment for syphilis. However, mercury had been in use since antiquity for the treatment of external (skin) conditions, and was employed at times to treat scabies. When syphilis appeared for the first time at the end of the fifteenth century, its presentation as a contagious pustular disease of the skin bore some resemblance to that of scabies. Thus, it was logical that mercury would be tried as a treatment for syphilis (143).

2. Friedman credits the Prussian Surgeon Jasser (14, 88).

3. von Hebra wrote: 'Medical writers and hospital surgeons have vied with each other in continually extolling the value of new ones [sulphur preparations] ... hitherto no reason has been shown for preferring one of them to another.'

4. Cazenave was incidentally the first person to describe the clinical features of the rheumatological disorder lupus (lupus érythémateux).

5. Hardy's treatment has also been described as follows:

   Every day patients with scabies were gathered in two bathrooms (men and women separately) in Hôpital Saint-Louis—a practice that endured until the 1970's. Each of them had to scrub the skin of the patient next to him with black soap for 20 minutes. Then he took a bath in lukewarm water for one hour, continuing to rub his skin.

   Afterwards a sulphur-potash-lard concoction was applied, and the patient was allowed to dress but told to leave on the medicine for 4–5 hours (157).

6. A variety of arthropods have acquired pyrethroid resistance through the development of mutations in their voltage-sensitive sodium channels (Vssc). Similar findings have been detected in *Sarcoptes scabiei*. Under select experimental conditions, dogs with a high canine-scabies burden who have been continually exposed to permethrin have been shown to develop permethrin-resistant mites. DNA sequencing of these permethrin-resistant canine scabies mites shows similar mutations in their voltage-sensitive sodium channels (Vssc) as seen in other pyrethroid-resistant arthropods (207).

7. A 1997 study reported that there was an increased number of deaths in elderly patients residing at a long term care facility who were treated with ivermectin (13), though other studies did not support this finding (154). A recent reassessment of the original study has revealed methodological flaws, and ivermectin is generally accepted as being safe in all age categories. In spite of this, however, some physicians continue to be wary about prescribing ivermectin for the elderly (155).

8. Specifically, ivermectin is thought to act on glutamate-gated chloride ion channels, and secondarily on gamma-aminobutyric acid-gated chloride ion channels (26).

9. For lesions to be defined as typical, within the same anatomical area three or more 2–3 mm red bumps (papules) must be present. In areas of skin that encompass body folds, typical lesions can sometimes be larger. In adults the typical distribution of lesions is along the circle of Hebra, as previously described. In infants typical distribution is also defined to include lesions on the head and scalp (156).

10. In tropical settings, topical medications should also be applied to face and scalp.

9

Conclusion

Mrs. Stein

Rhonda popped her head in my office. 'Your 3 o'clock, Mrs. Stein, is roomed. She's with her son, who says she is scratching herself to pieces.' With an introduction like that, the case could be pretty much anything—eczema, psoriasis, a medication side-effect, or even a cutaneous manifestation of an underlying medical illness. But of course my scabies antenna immediately perked up. I entered the room and introduced myself. Poor Mrs. Stein was wheelchair bound and quiet. She must have been in her early nineties. 'She doesn't say much', her son chimed in, 'but boy does she scratch.' Poor Mrs. Stein had scabs all along her arms, belly, and waistline. But no burrows, or at least none that I could appreciate. I obtained some more history from her son, examined her closely, and decided to take a scraping from the crusted areas on her arm. Mrs. Stein didn't exactly appreciate my scratching her up with a scalpel, but also didn't seem to have much energy to move away or even express her displeasure. Certainly, demographically she fell into a higher than average risk profile. Yet a trip with my scrapings to the microscope didn't show anything noteworthy.

I suppose missing the diagnosis of scabies, which I have undoubtedly done in the past, isn't the worst thing a dermatologist can do. I suppose I could have made my best guess and prescribed Mrs. Stein and her son scabies therapy empirically. But after years in practice I am now much more tenacious. If a patient has scabies, I want to document and prove it. If I don't, then who ever will? After all, I find it so much more satisfying to know exactly what I am treating. So, I went back to re-examine Mrs. Stein, and performed two additional rounds of scraping, both negative.

Frustrated, I took a moment to collect my thoughts. Poor Mrs. Stein. In spite of all my readings, downloading of papers, hunting down old manuscripts, in spite of my bizarre fascination with this historical disease, I couldn't tell you for sure if she even had it. I had professionally grown up and was now the authority. There was no Dr N. to turn to for help. And then suddenly, it dawned on me... Back I went to Mrs. Stein, who hadn't moved in the slightest. I picked up her hands, proceeded to take a small scraping of the greasy detritus under her fingernails, and smeared it on a glass slide. There under the microscope was a sickly looking shrivelled mite, replete with its hideous spines.

I looked up and Rhonda was peering over at me, wondering why I kept on going back to the microscope. 'Scabies', I mouthed. Her jaw dropped. 'Close down the room?' she whispered. Just then I had visions of Mellanby's volunteers stripping down and jumping under the blankets of known scabietic patients, trying and repeatedly failing to contract the disease themselves. 'Guess what?' I replied most assuredly. 'No need to bother.'

References

1. M. Hicks and D. Elston. Scabies. Dermatologic Therapy, 22 (4), July–Aug 2009, 279–92.
2. K. Mellanby. Scabies in 1976. Royal Society of Health Journal, 97 (1), Feb 1977, 32–6.
3. D. Mimouni et al. Seasonality Trends of Scabies in a Young Adult Population: A 20-Year Follow-up. British Journal of Dermatology, 149 (1), July 2003, 157–9.
4. D. Hogan et al. Diagnosis and Treatment of Childhood Scabies and Pediculosis. Pediatric Clinics of North America, 38 (4), Aug 1991, 941–57.
5. U. Hengge et al. Scabies: A Ubiquitous Neglected Skin Disease. The Lancet Infectious Diseases, 6 (12), Dec 2006, 769–79.
6. F. Knowles. Scabies in Military and Civil Life. Journal of the American Medical Association, 70 (20), 1918, 1657–8.
7. T. Meinking. Infestations. Current Problems in Dermatology, 11 (3), May–June 1999, 103–14.
8. B. Heilesen. Studies on *Acarus scabiei* and Scabies. Supplementum XIV (Vol XXVI) Acta Dermato-Venereologica, 1946.
9. L. Arlian et al. Survival and Infestivity of *Sarcoptes scabiei var. canis* and *var. hominis*. Journal of the American Academy of Dermatology, 11 (2 Pt 1), Aug 1984, 210–15.
10. J. Alexander. Scabies and Pediculosis. The Practitioner, 200 (199), May 1968, 632–44.
11. S. Estes and L. Arlian. Survival of *Sarcoptes scabiei*. Journal of the American Academy of Dermatology, 5 (3), Sept 1981, 343.
12. R. Carslaw et al. Mites in the Environment of Cases of Norwegian Scabies. British Journal of Dermatology, 92 (3), Mar 1975, 333–7.
13. R. Barkwell and S. Shields. Deaths Associated with Ivermectin Treatment of Scabies. The Lancet, 349 (9059), Apr 1997, 1144–5.
14. R. Friedman. The Story of Scabies. Froben Press, 1947.
15. K. Mellanby. Scabies. E. W. Classey Ltd., 1972.
16. J. Lane. Bonomo's Letter to Redi. Archives of Dermatology and Syphilology, 18 (1), July 1928, 1–25.
17. D. Montgomery. The Strange History of the Vesicle in Scabies. Annals of Medical History, 1937, 219–29.
18. R. Mead. An Abstract of a Letter from Dr. Bonomo to Signior Redi Containing some Observations Concerning the Worms of Humane Bodies. Philosophical Transactions, 23, Jan– Feb 1703, 1296–9.
19. K. Mellanby. Human Guinea Pigs, London, Merlin Press 1945 (then 1973). Reprinted in 2020 as L.M. Rasmussen (ed) Human Guinea Pigs, by Kenneth Mellanby, A Reprint with Commentaries. Philosophy and Medicine, 134, Springer Nature Switzerland AG, 2020.
20. G. Pernet. Historical Notes on Scabies, with Remarks on the Palaeontology of the Acarus. British Journal of Dermatology, 37 (7), July 1925, 312–16.
21. R. Friedman. The Emperor's Itch. Froben Press, 1940.
22. JWR Munro. Report of Scabies Investigation. Journal of the Royal Army Medical Corps, 33, 1919, 1–41.

23. H. MacCormac and W. Small. The Scabies Problem on Active Service. British Medical Journal, 2 (2960), Sept 1917, 384–6.

24. J. Crissey and L. Parish. Ferdinand Hebra: A Reexamination of His Contributions to Dermatology. International Journal of Dermatology, 19 (10), Dec 1980, 585–8.

25. D. Elston. Controversies Concerning the Treatment of Lice and Scabies. Journal of the American Academy of Dermatology, 46 (5), May 2002, 794–6.

26. B. Currie and J. McCarthy. Permethrin and Ivermectin for Scabies. New England Journal of Medicine, 362 (8), Feb 2010, 717–24.

27. F. von Hebra. On Diseases of the Skin, Vol 2. New Sydenham Society, 1868.

28. M. Svartman et al. Epidemic Scabies and Acute Glomerulonephritis in Trinidad. The Lancet, 1 (7744), Jan 1972, 249–51.

29. A. Madsen. Why Acarus scabiei Avoids the Face. Acta Dermato-Venereologica, 45 (2), 1965, 167–8.

30. R. Cabrera et al. The Immunology of Scabies. Seminars in Dermatology, 12 (1), Mar 1993, 15–21.

31. M. Green. Epidemiology of Scabies. Epidemiologic Reviews, 11, 1989, 126–50.

32. E. Danopoulos et al. Serious Poisoning by Hexachlorocyclohexane. American Medical Association Archives of Industrial Hygiene and Occupational Medicine, 8 (6), 1953, 582–7.

33. R. Wolf and B. Davidovici. Treatment of Scabies and Pediculosis: Facts and Controversies. Clinics in Dermatology, 28 (5), Sept–Oct 2010, 511–18.

34. D. Taplin et al. A Comparative Trial of Three Treatment Schedules for the Eradication of Scabies. Journal of the American Academy of Dermatology, 9 (4), Oct 1983, 550–4.

35. V. Usha and T. Nair. A Comparative Study of Oral Ivermectin and Topical Permethrin Cream in the Treatment of Scabies. Journal of the American Academy of Dermatology, 42 (2 Pt 1), Feb 2000, 236–40.

36. N. Scheinfeld. Controlling Scabies in Institutional Settings: a Review of Medications, Treatment Models, and Implementation. American Journal of Clinical Dermatology, 5 (1), 2004, 31–7.

37. J. Heukelbach and H Feldmeier. Scabies. The Lancet, 367 (9524), May 2006, 1767–74.

38. S. Walton and B. Currie. Problems in Diagnosing Scabies, a Global Disease in Human and Animal Populations. Clinical Microbiology Reviews, 20 (2), Apr 2007, 268–79.

39. Recent Researches on Scabies. The British and Foreign Medico-Chirurgical Review, (36), July–Oct 1865, 23–35.

40. B. Currie et al. First Documentation of In Vivo and In Vitro Ivermectin Resistance in Sarcoptes scabiei. Clinical Infectious Diseases, 39 (1), July 2004, e8–12.

41. J. Pemberton. Medical Experiments Carried out in Sheffield on Conscientious Objectors to Military Service During the 1939-45 War. International Journal of Epidemiology, 35 (3), June 2006, 556–8.

42. K. Mounsey et al. A Tractable Experimental Model for Study of Human and Animal Scabies. PLoS Neglected Tropical Diseases, 4 (7), July 2010, e756.

43. S. Walton et al. Acaricidal Activity of Melaleuca alternifolia (Tea Tree) Oil: In Vitro Sensitivity of Sarcoptes scabiei var. hominis to Terpinen-4-ol. Archives of Dermatology, 140 (5), May 2004, 563–6.

44. D. Taplin and T. Meinking. Pyrethrins and Pyrethroids in Dermatology. Archives of Dermatology, 126 (2), Feb 1990, 213–21.

45. A. Singal and G. Thami. Lindane Neurotoxicity in Childhood. American Journal of Therapeutics, 13 (3), May–June 2006, 277–80.

46. J. Witkowski and L. Parish. Scabies. Subungual Areas Harbor Mites. Journal of the American Medical Association, 252 (10), Sept 1984, 1318–9.

47. D. Van Neste. Human Scabies in Perspective. International Journal of Dermatology, 27 (1), Jan–Feb 1988, 10–15.

48. A. Kissmeyer. Rapid Ambulatory Treatment of Scabies with a Benzyl Benzoate Lotion. The Lancet, Jan 1937, 21.

49. E. Epstein. Trends in Scabies. American Medical Association Archives of Dermatology, 71 (2), Feb 1955, 192–6.

50. G. McLaughlin. History of Pyrethrum. In Pyrethrum: The Natural Insecticide. J. Casida (Ed), Academic Press, 1973, 3–15.

51. V. Jimenez-Lucho et al. Role of Prolonged Surveillance in the Eradication of Nosocomial Scabies in an Extended Care Veterans Affairs Medical Center. American Journal of Infection Control, 23 (1), Feb 1995, 44–9.

52. J. Sullivan et al. Successful Use of Ivermectin in the Treatment of Endemic Scabies in a Nursing Home. Australasian Journal of Dermatology, 38 (3), 1997, 137–40.

53. T. Davies et al. DDT, Pyrethrins, Pyrethroids, and Insect Sodium Channels. International Union of Biochemistry and Molecular Biology Life, 59 (3), Mar 2007, 151–62.

54. T. Cropley. The "Army Itch": A Dermatological Mystery of the American Civil War. Journal of the American Academy of Dermatology, 55 (2), Aug 2006, 302–8.

55. T. Meinking. The Treatment of Scabies with Ivermectin. New England Journal of Medicine, 333 (1), July 1995, 26–30.

56. M. Montesu and F. Cottoni. G.C. Bonomo and D. Cestoni. Discoverers of the Parasitic Origin of Scabies. American Journal of Dermatopathology, 13 (4), Aug 1991, 425–7.

57. L. Arlian et al. Cross Infestivity of *Sarcoptes scabiei*. Journal of the American Academy of Dermatology, 10 (6), June 1984, 979–85.

58. K. Mellanby. The Development of Symptoms, Parasitic Infection and Immunity in Human Scabies. Parasitology, 35 (4), Mar 1944, 197–206.

59. L. Arlian. Biology, Host Relations, And Epidemiology of *Sarcoptes Scabiei*. Annual Review of Entomology, 34, 1989, 139–61.

60. J. Alexander. Arthropods and the Human Skin, Springer-Verlag, 1984.

61. W. Campbell. Ivermectin, An Antiparasitic Agent. Medicinal Research Reviews, 13 (1), 1993, 61–79.

62. S. Walton et al. Scabies: New Future for a Neglected Disease. Advances in Parasitology, 57, 2004, 310–60.

63. W. Campbell. The Genesis of the Antiparasitic Drug Ivermectin. In Inventive Minds. R.J. Weber and D.N. Perkins (Eds), Oxford University Press, 194–214.

64. A. Lyell. Diagnosis and Treatment of Scabies. British Medical Journal, Apr 1967, 223–5.

65. S. Walton et al. Genetically Distinct Dog-Derived and Human-Derived *Sarcoptes Scabiei* in Scabies-Endemic Communities in Northern Australia. The American Journal of Tropical Medicine and Hygiene, 61 (4), Oct 1999, 542–7.

66. G. Argenziano et al. Epiluminescence Microscopy. A New Approach to In Vivo Detection of *Sarcoptes scabiei*. Archives of Dermatology, 133 (6), June 1997, 751–3.

67. M. Pacque et al. Pregnancy Outcome after Inadvertent Ivermectin Treatment During Community-Based Distribution. The Lancet, 336 (8729), Dec 1990, 1486–9.

68. M. Pacque et al. Community-Based Treatment of Onchocerciasis with Ivermectin: Safety, Efficacy, and Acceptability of Yearly Treatment. Journal of Infectious Disease, 163 (2), Feb 1991, 381–5.

69. R. Sharma et al. An Epidemiological Study of Scabies in a Rural Community in India. Annals of Tropical Medicine and Parasitology, 78 (2), Apr 1984, 157–64.

70. T. Cropley. The "Army Itch": Scabies in the American Civil War. The Society of Civil War Surgeons, Inc., 9 (3), July–Sept 2005, 65–8.

71. V. Sehgal et al. Scabies: A Study of Incidence and a Treatment Method. International Journal of Dermatology, 11 (2), Apr–June 1972, 106–11.

72. L. Arlian et al. Survival of Adult and Developmental Stages of Sarcoptes scabiei var. canis When Off the Host. Experimental and Applied Acarology, 6 (3), Apr 1989, 181–7.

73. L. Arlian and D. Vyszenski-Moher. Life Cycle of Sarcoptes scabiei var. canis. Journal of Parasitology, 74 (3), June 1988, 427–30.

74. A. Fain. Epidemiological Problems of Scabies. International Journal of Dermatology, 17 (1), Jan–Feb 1978, 20–30.

75. P. Glaziou et al. Comparison of Ivermectin and Benzyl Benzoate for Treatment of Scabies. Trop Medicine and Parasitology, 44 (4), Dec 1993, 331–2.

76. C. Johnson and K. Mellanby. The Parasitology of Human Scabies. Parasitology, 34 (3–4), 1942, 285–90.

77. J. Pringle. Observations on the Diseases of the Army in Camp and Garrison, 2nd ed. A Millar, D Wilson, T Durham, T Payne Publishers, 1753, 301–6.

78. A. Paller. Scabies in Infants and Small Children. Seminars in Dermatology, 12 (1), Mar 1993, 3–8.

79. W. Shelley and M. Wood. Larval Papule as a Sign of Scabies. Journal of the American Medical Association, 236 (10), Sept 1976, 1144–5.

80. C. Finnerud. Ferdinand Von Hebra and the Vienna School of Dermatology. American Medical Association Archives of Dermatology and Syphilology, 66 (2), Aug 1952, 223–32.

81. A. Dhana et al. Ivermectin Versus Permethrin in the Treatment of Scabies: A Systematic Review and Meta-Analysis of Randomized Controlled Trials. Journal of the American Academy of Dermatology, 78 (1), Jan 2018, 194–8.

82. C. Buck. Acupuncture and Chinese Medicine: Roots of Modern Practice. Singing Dragon, 2015.

83. C.E.P. Sixty Years Ago Scabies. Journal of the Royal Army Medical Corps, 117, 1971, 151–2.

84. J. White. Scabies. Boston Medical and Surgical Journal, 71 (22), 29 Dec 1864, 429–40.

85. K. Mellanby et al. The Treatment of Scabies. British Medical Journal, 4, July 1942, 1–4.

86. W. Wooldridge. The Gamma Isomer of Hexachlorocyclohexane in the Treatment of Scabies. Journal of Investigative Dermatology, 10 (5), May 1948, 363–6.

87. L. Saunders. Derris Root Treatment of Scabies. British Medical Journal, 1 (4190), 26 Apr 1941, 624–6.

88. G. Fischer. Surgery One Hundred Years Ago An Historical Study. Journal of the American Medical Association, 29 (10), Sept 1897, 481–2.

89. L. Romani et al. Mass Drug Administration for Scabies Control in a Population with Endemic Disease. New England Journal of Medicine, 373 (24), Dec 2015, 2305–13.

90. R. Sharma and A. Singal. Topical Permethrin and Oral Ivermectin in the Management of Scabies: A Prospective, Randomized, Double Blind, Controlled Study. Indian Journal of Dermatology, Venereology, and Leprosy, 77 (5), Sept–Oct 2011, 581–6.

91. B. Currie. Scabies and Global Control of Neglected Tropical Diseases. New England Journal of Medicine, 373 (24), Dec 2015, 2371–2.

92. D. Engelman et al. Consensus Criteria for the Diagnosis of Scabies: A Delphi Study of International Experts. PLOS Neglected Tropical Diseases, 12 (5), May 2018, 1–9.

93. GDB 2015 Disease and Injury Incidence and Prevalence Collaborators. Global, Regional, and National Incidence, Prevalence, and Years Lived with Disability for 310 Diseases and Injuries, 1990-2015: A Systematic Analysis for the Global Burden of Disease Study 2015. The Lancet, 388 (10053), Oct 2016, 1545–602.

94. M. Ameen et al. Oral Ivermectin for Treatment of Pediculosis Capitis. Pediatric Infectious Disease Journal, 29 (11), Nov 2010, 991–3.

95. C. Prins et al. Dermoscopy for the In vivo Detection of *Sarcoptes scabiei*. Dermatology, 208 (3), 2004, 241–3.

96. W. Shoop. Ivermectin Resistance. Parasitology Today, 9 (5), May 1993, 154–9.

97. P. Glaziou et al. Efficacy of Ivermectin for the Treatment of Head Lice. Tropical Medicine and Parasitology, 45 (3), Sept 1994, 253–4.

98. S. Rosumeck et al. Ivermectin and Permethrin for Treating Scabies (Review). Cochrane Database of Systematic Reviews, 4 (4), Apr 2018, 1–95.

99. D. Engelman et al. Toward the Global Control of Human Scabies: Introducing the International Alliance for the Control of Scabies. PLOS Neglected Tropical Diseases, 7 (8), Aug 2013, 1–4.

100. L. Romani et al. Prevalence of Scabies and Impetigo Worldwide: A Systematic Review. The Lancet Infectious Diseases, 15 (8), Aug 2015, 960–7.

101. W. Shelley and E.D. Shelley. Scanning Electron Microscopy of the Scabies Burrow and its Contents, with Special Reference to the *Sarcoptes scabiei* Egg. Journal American Academy of Dermatology, 9 (5), Nov 1983, 673–9.

102. W. Shelley et al. *Staphylococcus aureus* Colonization of Burrows in Erythrodermic Norwegian Scabies: A Case Study of Iatrogenic Contagion. Journal American Academy of Dermatology, 19 (4), Oct 1988, 673–8.

103. E. Nionaka et al. Scanning Electron Microscopic Observation of *Sarcoptes scabiei var. hominis*. Journal of Cutaneous Pathology, 12 (5), Oct 1985, 400–3.

104. M. Fimiani et al. The Behavior of *Sarcoptes scabiei var. hominis* in Human Skin: An Ultrastructural Study. Journal of Submicroscopic Cytology and Pathology, 29 (1), Jan 1997, 105–13.

105. W. Cunningham. The Artful Acarus. Scabies Exposed. New York Medical Journal, 102, 1915, 1042–5.

106. S. Rosumeck et al. Evaluation of Ivermectin vs Permethrin for Treating Scabies— Summary of a Cochrane Review. Journal of the American Medical Association Dermatology, 155 (6), June 2019, 730–2.

107. J. White. On the Increasing Prevalence of Scabies with Remarks upon Treatments. Boston Medical and Surgical Journal, 120, Feb 1889, 157–9.

108. K. Mellanby. Itching to Study Lice and Mites. The Scientist, 2 (8), May 1988.

109. A. Sakula. Joseph Skoda 1805-81: A Centenary Tribute to a Pioneer of Thoracic Medicine. Thorax, 36 (6), June 1981, 404–11.

110. H. Stelwagon. A Treatise on Diseases of the Skin, 8th ed. W.B. Saunders Company, 1918, 1243–51.

111. H. Stelwagon. Increasing Prevalence of Scabies. The Medical News, 63 (13), Sept 1893, 341–4.

112. F. Painter. Notes on Scabies in Boston. Boston Medical and Surgical Journal, 171 (2), July 1914, 54–8.

113. L. Romani et al. Mass Drug Administration for Scabies—2 Years Follow-up. New England Journal of Medicine, 381 (2), July 2019, 186–7.

114. E. Yew. Medical Inspection of Immigrants at Ellis Island, 1891-1924. Bulletin of the New York Academy of Medicine, 56 (5), June 1980, 488–510.

115. B. Terry et al. *Sarcoptes scabiei* Infestation Among Children in a Displacement Camp in Sierra Leone. Public Health, 115 (3), May 2001, 208–11.

116. B. Chadwick. George Washington's War. Sourcebooks, 2004.

117. B. Sokoloff. Napoleon. A Doctor's Biography. Prentice-Hall, 1937.

118. L. Sefton. Some Experiences in a Skin Department of a Prisoner-of-War Camp Hospital in Singapore 1942-5 Part II. The British Journal of Dermatology and Syphilis, 59 (4-5), Apr–May 1947, 159–68.

119. Obituaries. Prof J.W. Munro. Nature, 218, May 1968, 610–11.

120. B. Currie and U. Hengge. Scabies. In Tropical Dermatology, 2nd ed. S. Tyring, O. Lupi, and U. Hengge (Eds), Elsevier Press, 2017, 376–86.

121. J. Cassell et al. Scabies Outbreaks in Ten Care Homes for Elderly People: A Prospective Study of Clinical Features, Epidemiology, and Treatment Outcomes. The Lancet Infectious Diseases, 18 (8), Aug 2018, 894–902.

122. K. Mellanby. Biology of the Parasite. In Cutaneous Infestations and Insect Bites. M. Orkin and H. Maibach (Eds), Marcel Dekker, 1985, 13.

123. R. Friedman. The Story of Scabies-II. Medical Life, 41 (9), Sept 1934, 425–76.

124. R. Friedman. Johann Ernst Wichmann—The One Hundred and Fiftieth Anniversary of His Contribution to Scabies. Medical Life, 43, 1936, 171–210.

125. R. Friedman. The Story of Scabies. Medical Life, 41 (8), Aug 1934, 378–424.

126. H. Kiel. Scabies and the Queen Mab Passage in Romeo and Juliet. Journal of the History of Ideas, 18 (3), June 1957, 394–410.

127. E. Wilson. The Student's Book of Cutaneous Medicine and Diseases of the Skin. William Wood & Co, 1865. Proceedings of the Royal Society of Medicine.

128. H. MacCormac. Skin Diseases and their Treatment under War Conditions. Proceedings of the Royal Society of Medicine, 10 (Part 1), 1917, 120–56.

129. J. Crissey and L. Parish. The Dermatology and Syphilology of the Nineteenth Century. Praeger Publishers, 1981.

130. N.A. Richardson et al. Scabies outbreak management in refugee/migrant camps across Europe 2014–17: a retrospective qualitative interview study of healthcare staff experiences and perspectives. Preprint. 04/2021. https://doi.org/10.1101/2021.04.28.21256211

131. J. Degelau. Scabies in Long-Term Care Facilities. Infection Control and Hospital Epidemiology, 13 (7), July 1992, 421–5.

132. L. Arlian and M. Morgan. A Review of *Sarcoptes scabiei*: Past, Present and Future. Parasites & Vectors, 10 (297), June 2017, 1–22.

133. K. Holubar. Ferdinand von Hebra 1816-1880. On the Occasion of the Centenary of His Death. International Journal of Dermatology, 20 (4), May 1981, 291–5.

134. J. Cantrell. Scabies: Its Symptoms, Diagnosis, and Treatment. George S. Davis, 1893.

135. V. Robinson. Ferdinand Von Hebra Written on The Centenary of Hebra's Birth. Medical Review of Reviews, 22 (10), Oct 1916, 719–24.

136. J. Adams. Observations of Morbid Poisons Chronic and Acute, 2nd ed. J. Callow, 1807.

137. S. Graham. With Poor Immigrants to America. MacMillan Co, 1914.

138. K. Siena. The Moral Biology of 'The Itch' in Eighteenth-Century Britain. In A Medical History of Skin: Scratching the Surface. J. Reinarz and K. Siena (Eds), Pickering & Chatto, 2013.

139. D. Ghesquier. A Gallic Affair: The Case of the Missing Itch-Mite in French Medicine in the Early Nineteenth Century. Medical History, 43 (1), Jan 1999, 26–54.

140. M. DeLacy. The Germ of an Idea. Contagionism, Religion, and Society in Britain 1660-1730. Palgrave Macmillan, 2016.

141. W. Pusey. The History of Dermatology. Charles C. Thomas, 1933.

142. R. Mead. A Short Discourse Concerning Pestilential Contagion and Those Methods to Be Used to Prevent It. London, 1720.

143. O. Temkin. The Double Face of Janus and Other Essays in the History of Medicine. Johns Hopkins University Press, 1977.

144. M. DeLacy. Contagionism Catches On—Medical Ideology in Britain 1730-1800. Palgrave Macmillan, 2017.

145. B. Stoff et al. Expedited Partner Therapy for Scabies: Legal and Ethical Considerations. Journal of the American Academy of Dermatology, 69 (5), Nov 2013, 795–8.

146. J. Lester et al. Ethical Dilemmas and Legal Pitfalls in Prescribing for the Uninsured Indigent Patient: Reconciling the Irreconcilable. Journal of the American Academy of Dermatology, 68 (4), Apr 2013, 672–4.

147. R. Friedman. Bonomo and Cestoni: The Dispute Concerning Their Identity, the Authorship of the "Letter to Redi," and the Credit for the Discovery of the Acarian Origin of Scabies. In Abraham Levinson Anniversary Volume: Studies in Pediatrics and Medical History. S.R. Kagan (Ed), Froben Press, 1948, 279–96.

148. C. Singer. Notes on the Early History of Microscopy. Proceedings of the Royal Society of Medicine, 7 (Sect Hist Med), 1914, 247–79.

149. R. Friedman. Thomas Moffet: The Tercentenary of his Contribution to Scabies. Medical Life, 41 (1934), 620–35.

150. H. André. The True Identity of Pascal's Mite and the Diachronic Use of Ciron. Acarologia, 59 (2), 2019, 261–78.

151. T. Meinking et al. Infestations. In Pediatric Dermatology, 4th ed. L. Schachner and R. Hansen (Eds), Mosby Elsevier, 2011, 1556–74.

152. R. Roncalli. The History of Scabies in Veterinary and Human Medicine from Biblical to Modern Times. Veterinary Parasitology, 25 (2), July 1987, 193–8.

153. M. Levy et al. Ivermectin Safety in Infants and Children Under 15 kg Treated for Scabies: A Multicentric Observational Study. British Journal of Dermatology, 182 (4), Apr 2020, 1003–6.

154. R. Reintjes and C Hoek. Deaths Associated with Ivermectin for Scabies. The Lancet, 350 (9072), July 1997, 215.

155. J. Middleton et al. Ivermectin for the Control of Scabies Outbreaks in the UK. The Lancet, 394 (10214), Dec 2019, 2068–9.

156. D. Engelman et al. The 2020 International Alliance for the Control of Scabies: Consensus Criteria for the Diagnosis of Scabies. British Journal of Dermatology, 183 (5), Nov 2020, 808–20.

157. G. Tilles. Pierre Louis Phillipe Alfred Hardy. In Pantheon of Dermatology; Outstanding Historical Figures. C. Löser, G. Plewig, and W. Burgdorf (Eds.), Springer-Verlag Press, 2013, 438.

158. C. Bernigaud et al. How to Eliminate Scabies Parasites from Fomites: A High-Throughput Ex Vivo Experimental Study. Journal of the American Academy of Dermatology, 83 (1), July 2020, 241–5.

159. B. Beeson. Alibert. Archives of Dermatology and Syphilology, 26 (6), 1932, 1086–93.

160. D. Montgomery. Jean Louis Alibert. Archives of Dermatology and Syphilology, 19 (1), 1929, 89–97.

161. J.L. Alibert. Précis Théorique et Pratique sue Les Maladies de la Peau, 2nd ed. Paris, 1822.

162. La Polemica Bonomo—Lancisi sull' <<origine acarica della scabbia>>, Societa Italiana di Dermatologia E Sifilografia, Livorno, 1937.

163. M. Janier. Histoire du Sarcopte de la Gale. Histoire des Sciences Medicales, 28 (4), 1994, 365–79.

164. R. Friedman. "Scabies Day": June 20, 1937. Medical Life, 44 (3), Jan 1937, 229–51.

165. M. DeLacy and A. Cain. A Linnaean Thesis concerning Contagium Vivum: The 'Exanthemata Viva' of John Nyander and its Place in Contemporary Thought. Medical History, 39 (2), Apr 1995, 159–85.

166. R. Friedman. A Translation of Bonomo's Manuscript Letter to Redi. Medical Life, Mar 1937, 156–64.

167. R. Friedman. Zan-yun-fang (Ch'ao Yuan-fang): Discoverer of the Acarian Origin of Scabies? Medical Life, Sept 1937, 331–2.

168. C. Winslow. The Conquest of Epidemic Disease: A Chapter in the History of Ideas. Princeton University Press, 1943.

169. G. Scanni. The Mite-Gallery Unit: A New Concept for Describing Scabies through Entodermoscopy. Tropical Medicine and Infectious Disease, 4 (1), Mar 2019, 1–12.

170. Z. Klassen et al. Giovanni Maria Lancisi (1654-1720): Anatomist and Papal Physician. Clinical Anatomy, 24 (7), Oct 2011, 802–6.

171. U. Viviani. Un Errore del Gran Medico Aretino G.M. Lancisi. In Curiosita Storiche e Letterarie Aretine. 1921, 118–23.

172. S. Romero et al. The Stuff of Nightmares: Inside the Migrant Detention Center in Clint, Texas. El Paso Times and New York Times, 6 July 2019.

173. J. Munro. Pests of Stored Products. Hutchinson & Co, 1966.

174. B. Stanton et al. Scabies in Urban Bangladesh. Journal of Tropical Medicine and Hygiene, 90 (5), Oct 1987, 219–26.

175. R. Friedman. Carolus Musitanus. The 250th Anniversary of His Contribution to Scabies. Medical Life, 45, 1938, 177–87.

176. M. Elliott et al. A Photostable Pyrethroid. Nature, 246, Nov 1973, 169–70.

177. M. Nassif and O. Kamel. A Field Trial with Permethrin Against Bodylice *Pediculus humanus humanus* in Egypt, 1976. Pest Management Science, 8 (3), June 1977, 301–4.

178. D. Taplin and T Meinking. Pyrethrins and Pyrethroids for the Treatment of Scabies and Pediculosis. Seminars in Dermatology, 6 (2), June 1987, 125–35.

179. D. Taplin. Eradication of Scabies with a Single Treatment Schedule. Journal of the American Academy of Dermatology, 9 (4), Oct 1983, 546–50.

180. D. Taplin. Permethrin 5% Dermal Cream: A New Treatment for Scabies. Journal of the American Academy of Dermatology, 15 (5 Pt 1), Nov 1986, 995–1001.

181. O. Chosidow. Clinical practices. Scabies. New England Journal of Medicine, 354 (16), Apr 2006, 1718–27.

182. B. Beeson. *Acarus scabiei* Study of Its History. Archives of Dermatology and Syphilology, 16 (3), Sept 1927, 294–307.

183. J. Stokes. Scabies Among the Well-to-Do. Journal of the American Medical Association, Feb 1936, 674–8.

184. R. Hansen and P. Lynch. Scabies: Problems in Physician Recognition. Arizona Medicine, 33 (5), May 1976, 366–8.

185. M. Ramos-e-Silva. Giovan Cosimo Bonomo (1663–1696): Discoverer of the Etiology of Scabies. International Journal of Dermatology, 37 (8), Aug 1998: 625–30.

186. H. Feldmeier et al. The Epidemiology of Scabies in an Impoverished Community in Rural Brazil: Presence and Severity of Disease are Associated with Poor Living Conditions and Illiteracy. Journal of the American Academy of Dermatology, 60 (3), Mar 2009, 436–43.

187. E. Trice and R. Manson. Camp Itch: A Retrospective Study 100 Years Later. Southern Medical Journal, 59 (1), January 1996, 10–14.

188. M. Orkin and H. Maibach. Modern Aspects of Scabies. Current Problems in Dermatology, 13, 1985, 109–27.

189. M. Orkin and H. Maibach. Current Concepts in Parasitology: This Scabies Pandemic. New England Journal of Medicine, 298 (9), March 1978, 496–8.

190. J. Savin. Mellanby on Scabies. Clinical and Experimental Dermatology, 27 (1), Jan 2002, 86–7.

191. R. Wolf et al. Scabies: The Diagnosis of Atypical Cases. Cutis. 55 (6), June 1995, 370–1.

192. R. Scher. Subungual Scabies. American Journal of Dermatopathology, 5 (2), April 1983, 187–9.

193. M. Boffa et al. Lindane Neurotoxicity. British Journal of Dermatology, 133 (6), Dec 1995, 1013.

194. J. Hyde. Scabies in The United States of America and Canada. American Journal of the Medical Sciences, 129 (3), March 1905, 453–64.

195. K. Mellanby et al. Experiments of the Survival and Behaviour of the Itch Mite, Sarcoptes Scabiei DeG, var hominis. Bulletin of Entomological Research. 33 (4), Dec 1942, 267–71.

196. A. Crump. The Advent of Ivermectin: People, Partnerships, and Principles. Trends in Parasitology, 30 (9), Sept 2014, 423–5.

197. L. Kornblee and F. Combes. Gammexane in Treatment of Scabies. Archives of Dermatology and Syphilology, 61 (3), 1950 Mar, 407–12.

198. C. Cooper and M. Jackson. Outbreak of Scabies in a Small Community Hospital. American Journal of Infection Control, 14 (4), August 1986, 173–9.

199. A. Chang and L. Fuller. Scabies—An Ancient Disease with Unanswered Questions in Modern Times. Journal of the American Medical Association Dermatology, 154 (9), Sept 2018, 999–1000.

200. O. Temkin. Galenism: Rise and Decline of a Medical Philosophy. Cornell University Press, Ithaca and London, 1973.

201. L. Garcia-Ballester. Galen and Galenism: Theory and Medical Practice from Antiquity to the European Renaissance. Ashgate Publishing Ltd, 2002.

202. S. Walker et al. The Prevalence and Association with Health-Related Quality of Life of Tungiasis and Scabies in Schoolchildren in Southern Ethiopia. PLOS Neglected Tropical Diseases, 11 (8), Aug 2017, 1–11.

203. C. Thomas et al. Ectoparasites: Scabies. Journal of the American Academy of Dermatology, 82 (3), March 2020, 533–48.

204. J. Davis et al. A Novel Clinical Grading Scale to Guide the Management of Crusted Scabies. PLOS Neglected Tropical Diseases, 7 (9), Sept 2013, 1–5.

205. C. Wilson. The Invisible World: Early Modern Philosophy and the Invention of the Microscope. Princeton University Press, 1995.

206. R. Friedman. The Story of Scabies-IV: At Tabari:Discoverer of the Acarus scabiei. Medical Life, June 1938, 163–76.

207. C. Pasay. High-Resolution Melt Analysis for the Detection of a Mutation Associated with Permethrin Resistance in a Population of Scabies Mites. Medical and Veterinary Entomology, 22 (1), Mar 2008, 82–8.

208. S. Walton et al. Studies in vitro on the Relative Efficacy of Current Acaricides for Sarcoptes scabiei var. hominis. Transactions of the Royal Society of Tropical Medicine and Hygiene, 94 (1), Jan–Feb 2000, 92–6.

209. A. Crump et al. The Onchocerciasis Chronicle: From the Beginning to the End? Trends in Parasitology, 28 (7), July 2012, 280–8.
210. T Spooner. A Short Account of the Itch, 6th ed, J Roberts, 1728.
211. W. Campbell (Ed). *Ivermectin and Abamectin*. Springer-Verlag, 1989.
212. S. Veraldi et al. Why is the Back so Rarely Involved in Scabies? Giornale Italiano di Dermatologia e Venereologia, 155 (1), Feb 2020, 113–4.
213. C. Karimkhani et al. The Global Burden of Scabies: A Cross-Sectional Analysis from the Global Burden of Disease Study 2015. The Lancet Infectious Diseases, 17 (12), Dec 2017, 1247–54.

Index

For the benefit of digital users, indexed terms that span two pages (e.g., 52–53) may, on occasion, appear on only one of those pages.

Tables and figures are indicated by *t* and *f* following the page number

acarophobia 158
Adams, Joseph 114–15
akari 97, 115n.1
Alexander, John O'Donel 155–56
Alibert, Jean-Louis 121–24, 123*f*, 126
al-Tabari 95–96
American Civil War 84–85
ancient Greeks 93–94, 95
animalculism 113, 125
ankle lesions 45
Aristotle 93–94
armpit lesions 45
army itch 84–85
Avenzoar 96
avermectins 147
axilla lesions 45

back lesions 51
bacterial infection 79, 85–86
Balsam of Peru 141
Bazin, Pierre-Antoine-Ernest 138–39
bed-sharing 48–50, 78–79
Benedictus, Alexander 96–97
benzyl benzoate 141
blister 68–70, 69*f*, 97–98, 125
bloodletting 99
body humours 95, 98–99
body site predilection 40–51, 70
boils 85–86
Bonomo, Giovanni Cosimo 100–10,
 111–13, 141
bug bomb 144
burrows 13–14, 24–26, 29, 64–68
buttock lesions 45

camp itch 84–85
Cazenave, Pierre, Louis Alphee 138–39

Celsus, Aulus Cornelius 94, 137
Cestoni, Diacinto 100–10, 100*f*,
 111–13, 141
Ch'ao Yuan-fang 94
Chauliac, Guy de 96–97
children, scabies risk 77–78
chrysanthemum flowers 141, 143–44
circle of Hebra 45, 48*f*
cleanliness 16
close contacts
 transmission of scabies 32–33, 78
 treating 23–24, 31, 39, 156–57
conscientious objectors, research
 volunteers 10–13, 18
consensus criteria 153–55, 154*t*
crusted (Norwegian) scabies 34–36, 64,
 150, 151*f*, 152, 156
Cunningham, William 50–51

Dalmatian insect powder 143
deGeer, Charles 113–14
delta-winged jet sign 26
dementia 77–78
Demodex folliculorum 50–51
dermoscopy 6, 26, 28*f*
derris root 141
diagnosis of scabies 14–15, 24–31, 152–55
differential diagnosis 153*t*
dirt disease 16
disinfestation/disinfection 16–17, 33–34
drug-resistance 146, 152
drug treatment *see* treatment of scabies

elbow lesions 45, 50
elderly, scabies risk 77–78
Elimite *see* permethrin
epidemics *see* outbreaks of scabies

examination of patients 29
expedited partner therapy 52n.1
etymology 56–57

face lesions 50–51, 70
'Fairholmes', Sheffield 11
fingernail(s) 32, 35*f*, 36*f*, 51, 155–56, 161–62
fomite transmission 10, 16, 33–36,
    53n.6–7, 88
foot lesions 45, 50
Frank, Joseph 138
Franklin, Benjamin 83, 84*f*
Friedman, Reuben 50, 82, 89, 94,
    127*f*, 140–41

Galenism 113
Galès, Jean Chrysanthe 123–24
gammexane see *lindane*
genitalia *see* penis lesions
geriatric population 77–78
global burden of scabies 79
glomerulonephritis 79
Goodhue, Lyle 144

hand lesions 40, 48–50, 51
Hauptmann, August 98, 99*f*
head lesions 50–51, 70
Heilesen, Bjørn 48–51, 49*f*
herd immunity 73–74
hexachlorocyclohexane 141–42
Hildegarde, Saint 96
histopathology 66*f*
Hôpital Saint-Louis, Paris 121–22,
    122*f*, 138–39
humidity 33–34, 70
humours 95, 98–99, 111
hypersensitivity reaction 29, 157–58

iatromechanics 111
ichthyol ointment 86
immigration 81–82
immune response 68
immunosuppression 78
impetigo 79, 85–86
infants, scabies risk 77–78
ink test 26
in-vitro assay 86–87
institutional outbreaks 37–39, 150
International Alliance for the Control of
    Scabies, diagnostic criteria 152–55

itching 14, 29–31
    night-time 14, 29–31, 87
    postscabies 157–58
ivermectin 146–52, 151*f*
ivermectin-resistance potential 152

Johansson, Bert 80–81
Joubert, Laurent 96–97

kidney disease 79
knee lesions 50
Koch's postulates 115
Krebs, Sir Hans 17–18

Lancisi, Giovanni Maria 106–10, 107*f*
larval papules 29, 38, 62, 65*f*, 66*f*
Latreille, Pierre André 113–14
lindane 141–43
lindane resistance 145
Linnaeus, Carl 113–14
Lugol, Jean 124
Lyclear *see* permethrin

MacCormac, H. 85–86, 88
Mead, Richard 104–6, 104*f*, 110, 113
Mellanby, Kenneth 6–18, 7*f*, 19*f*, 140–41
    body site predilection 40, 51
    mass screening examination 15, 45
    scabies rash 29
    scabies transmission research 10–17
    sexual transmission of scabies 78–79
    shipwreck survival research 17
    vitamin deprivation studies 17–18
Mercuriale, Girolamo 98–99
mercury therapy 86, 136
microscopy 98, 101, 113
military personnel 10, 16–17, 74–
    76, 82–89
Mitchell, James 88
Moffet, Thomas 93–94, 97, 124
Munro, Captain J.W. 86–88
Musitanus, Carolus 118n.19, 124

needle extraction 87, 95, 96–97, 101,
    125–26, 136–37
night-time itch 14, 29–31, 87
nipple lesions 48–50
Nix *see* permethrin
Norwegian (crusted) scabies 34–36, 64,
    150, 151*f*, 152, 156

onchocerciasis 148–49
outbreaks of scabies
    cyclical 73–76
    institutional 37–39
    vulnerable populations 80–81

parasite rate 15
Pare, Ambrose 96–97
'peek-a-boo' examination 29
penis lesions 40, 45, 48–50, 88
permethrin 85, 141, 143–46
permethrin-resistance potential 146
Persian dust 143
petroleum 141–42
physical examination of patients 29
ping-pong transmission 31
postscabies pruritus 31, 157–58
poststreptococcal glomerulonephritis 79
poverty, scabies risk 78
Pringle, Sir John 83, 138
psychological effects of scabies 158
Pusey, William 110
pustule 68–70, 69f, 97–98, 125
pyrethrins 141, 143–45

quicksilver girdle 136

rash, distribution 29, 30f
Raspail, François Vincent 124–25
Redi, Francesco 100, 102–3, 102f
reinfestation 14, 32
Renucci, Simon François 115, 125–
    27, 126f
rheumatic heart disease 79
risk factors for scabies 77–79
river blindness 148–49
Romance of the Roses (poem) 96–97
Romans 94
rotenone 141
Rush, Benjamin 83

Sarcoptes scabiei (scabies mite)
    body site predilection 40–51, 70
    burrows 13–14, 24–26, 64–68
    cross-species infection 56–57
    derivation of name 56–57
    differential diagnosis 153t
    egg laying 61, 101–2
    female mites 14, 32, 57, 61, 62, 64–
        68, 70

first description 95–96, 100
first known sketch 98, 99f
larvae 61
lifecycle 32, 57–62
male mites 57–61, 62
mating habits 57–61, 63f
moulting pouch 62
naming by Latreille 113–14
nymphs 62
parasite rate 15
phylogeny 56–57
physical appearance 57
regional names for afflictions 98–99
scanning electron microscopy 58f
size 57
transplantation experiments 14, 87
scabies mite see Sarcoptes scabiei
'scabies station' 128–30
Scaliger, Julius Caesar 96–97
Schönlein, Johann Lucas 127
Schwiebe, Jacob 110–11
scratching 29, 32, 51, 79, 131
screening examination 45
scrotum lesions 45, 48–50
scybala 24–26, 67f
sensitization 13–14, 29–31, 32
seven-year itch 74–76
Seven Year's (Silesian) War 74–76
sexual transmission 78–79
Shakespeare, William (Romeo and
    Juliet) 96–97
Sheffield 11
shipwreck research 17
skin scrapings 24–26, 29, 55–56
Skoda, Joseph 128–29, 130
Sloane, Hans 113
Small, W.D. 85–86
soab 96
socioeconomic risk factors 78
spontaneous generation 95, 101–3
Spooner, Thomas 99, 132–33n.13, 136,
    137, 157
staphylococcal bacteria 79
Stelwagon, H.W. 81–82
Stokes, John 24
'stoving' 16–17
streptococcal bacteria 79
Sullivan, William 144
sulphur treatment 85, 94, 137–41
suspected scabies see consensus criteria

tea tree oil 141
Thibierge, Georges 89
tobacco leaf treatment 141
transmission of scabies
    bed-sharing 48–50, 78–79
    close contacts 31, 32–33, 78
    fomites 33–36, 88
    Mellanby's research 10–17
    ping-pong 31
    sexual contact 78–79
treatment of scabies
    Balsam of Peru 141
    benzyl benzoate 141
    bloodletting 99
    chrysanthemum flowers 141, 143
    close contacts 23–24, 31, 39, 156–57
    correct application of topical
        treatment 155–56
    derris root 141
    drug-resistant scabies 146, 152
    English method 138–39
    experimental natural products 85, 141
    failure of treatment 152–58
    ichthyol 86
    ivermectin 146–52
    lindane 141–43
    at Mellanby's hospital 14–15
    mercury 86, 136
    modified English method 139
    needle extraction 95, 96–97, 101,
        125–26, 136–37

permethrin 85, 141, 143–46, 150
petroleum 141–42
pregnancy 140–41, 152
pyrethrins 141, 143–45
'rapid treatment' 139
rotenone 141
sulphur 85, 94, 137–41
tea tree oil 141
tobacco leaf 141
Vlemingkx's method 139
written instructions 156
tropical scabies 33–34, 70, 79, 151

van Helmont, Jan Baptiste 110–11
Vivani, Ugo 110
von Hebra, Ferdinand Ritter 29, 50, 78, 85,
    128–31, 129f, 138–39, 140

wartime scabies 10, 74–76, 82–89
White, James 51
Wichmann, Johann Ernst 75, 114
Wiener Allgemeines
    Krankenhaus 130
Wilson, Erasmus 140–41
World War I 85–89
World War II 10
wrist lesions 40, 48–50

Yandell, Lunsford Pitts Jr. 84–85

zaraath 93